SpringerBriefs in Statistics

JSS Research Series in Statistics

The current research of statistics in Japan has expanded in several directions in line with recent trends in academic activities in the area of statistics and statistical sciences over the globe. The core of these research activities in statistics in Japan has been the Japan Statistical Society (JSS). This society, the oldest and largest academic organization for statistics in Japan, was founded in 1931 by a handful of pioneer statisticians and economists and now has a history of about 80 years. Many distinguished scholars have been members, including the influential statistician Hirotugu Akaike, who was a past president of JSS, and the notable mathematician Kiyosi Itô, who was an earlier member of the Institute of Statistical Mathematics (ISM), which has been a closely related organization since the establishment of ISM. The society has two academic journals: the Journal of the Japan Statistical Society (English Series) and the Journal of the Japan Statistical Society (Japanese Series). The membership of JSS consists of researchers, teachers, and professional statisticians in many different fields including mathematics, statistics, engineering, medical sciences, government statistics, economics, business, psychology, education, and many other natural, biological, and social sciences. The JSS Series of Statistics aims to publish recent results of current research activities in the areas of statistics and statistical sciences in Japan that otherwise would not be available in English; they are complementary to the two JSS academic journals, both English and Japanese. Because the scope of a research paper in academic journals inevitably has become narrowly focused and condensed in recent years, this series is intended to fill the gap between academic research activities and the form of a single academic paper. The series will be of great interest to a wide audience of researchers, teachers, professional statisticians, and graduate students in many countries who are interested in statistics and statistical sciences, in statistical theory, and in various areas of statistical applications.

More information about this subseries at http://www.springer.com/series/13497

Osamu Komori · Shinto Eguchi

Statistical Methods for Imbalanced Data in Ecological and Biological Studies

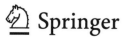 Springer

Osamu Komori
Seikei University
Musashino, Tokyo, Japan

Shinto Eguchi
The Institute of Statistical Mathematics
Tachikawa, Tokyo, Japan

ISSN 2191-544X   ISSN 2191-5458   (electronic)
SpringerBriefs in Statistics
ISSN 2364-0057   ISSN 2364-0065   (electronic)
JSS Research Series in Statistics
ISBN 978-4-431-55569-8   ISBN 978-4-431-55570-4   (eBook)
https://doi.org/10.1007/978-4-431-55570-4

This Springer imprint is published by the registered company Springer Japan KK part of Springer Nature. The registered company address is: Shiroyama Trust Tower, 4-3-1 Toranomon, Minato-ku, Tokyo 105-6005, Japan

Preface

This book is new in two main ways. In Chap. 1, it provides a recent review of challenging in prediction and classification caused by imbalanced data, and in the later chapters, it introduces several of the latest statistical methods for dealing with these problems. We discuss data imbalances from two points of view. The first is quantitative imbalance, in which the sample size in one population greatly outnumbers that in another population; this is investigated in Chap. 2 using fishery data sets. In Chap. 3, as an extreme case of imbalance, we discuss presence-only data, in which the presence of a species has been confirmed, but information about absence is indecisive; this is especially common in ecology in predictions of habitat distribution. The second is qualitative imbalance (in Chap. 4), in which the data distribution of one population can be well specified, whereas that of another is highly heterogeneous. A typical example is the existence of outliers in gene expression data, and another is the heterogeneous characteristics often observed in the case group in case-control studies. In Chap. 5, we introduce several machine learning methods to deal with imbalanced high-dimensional data sets. In these chapters, we discuss extensions of logistic regression models, Fisher's linear discriminant analysis, Maxent, AdaBoost, and AUCBoost for imbalanced data, thereby providing a novel framework for the improvement of prediction, classification, and performance of variable selection. The weights of data or objective functions in these methods play important roles in alleviating data imbalances. This book also provides applications of the proposed methods to real data sets using the statistical software R.

Finally, we would like to express our gratitude toward Prof. Tomonari Sei of the University of Tokyo for his careful and detailed comments on our manuscript.

Tokyo, Japan

Osamu Komori
Shinto Eguchi

Contents

Chapter 1
Introduction to Imbalanced Data

Abstract An imbalance of sample sizes among class labels makes it difficult to obtain high classification accuracy in many scientific fields, including medical diagnosis, bioinformatics, biology, and fisheries management. This difficulty is referred to as "class imbalance problem" and is considered to be among the 10 most important problems in data mining research. This topic has also been widely discussed in several machine learning workshops. The critical feature of the imbalance problem is that it significantly degrades the performance of standard classification methods, which implicitly assume balanced class distributions and equal costs of misclassification for each class. Hence, new strategies are required for mitigating such imbalances, based on resampling techniques, modification of the classification algorithms, adjustment of weights for class distributions, and so on.

Keywords Evaluation measures · Imbalance · Over-sampling · Under-sampling

1.1 Sampling Strategies

A simple way to deal with the imbalance problem is to increase the sample size of data in minority class ($y = 1$) by resampling, or to decrease it in the majority class ($y = 0$) by removing redundant observations. These techniques are referred to as over-sampling and under-sampling, respectively. However, random over-sampling is prone to result in overfitting to the augmented data, whereas random under-sampling is also likely to remove observations that are important to classification performance. Hence, several methods for improving over- or under- sampling techniques have been proposed. In the following, we assume that observations x_0 and x_1 come from the population of class 0 ($y = 0$) and class 1 ($y = 1$), respectively.

© The Author(s), under exclusive licence to Springer Japan KK 2019
O. Komori and S. Eguchi, *Statistical Methods for Imbalanced Data in Ecological and Biological Studies*, JSS Research Series in Statistics,
https://doi.org/10.1007/978-4-431-55570-4_1

1.1.1 Under-Sampling Techniques

1.1.1.1 Tomek Link

A pair (x_0, x_1) is called a Tomek link [12] if it holds for any observation z that

$$d(x_0, x_1) \leq d(x_0, z) \text{ and } d(x_0, x_1) \leq d(z, x_1), \qquad (1.1)$$

where $d(x_0, x_1)$ is the distance between x_0 and x_1. A Tomek link can detect outliers or observations near a boundary between distributions of $y = 0$ and $y = 1$ as shown in Fig. 1.1. Panel (a) shows the distribution of the original data with observations from $y = 0$ (majority class) and $y = 1$ (minor class) denoted by black circles and red crosses, respectively. In panel (b), the Tomek links are shown as blue line segments. In panel (c), observations in the majority class identified as Tomek links have been removed. Similarly, in panel (d), observations identified as Tomek links in both classes have been removed. This practice is referred to as data cleaning [11]. In (c) and (d), the surrounding area is cleaned, which would improve the classification accuracy in some situations. In (b), an observation of $y = 1$ above the boundary is not identified as a Tomek link. This is because the area around the observation is sparse, which is closely related to the difficulty of classification with imbalanced data [2, 9]. By finding Tomek links, we can detect prototypes, which are a subset of the whole data set and regarded as useful for classification.

1.1.1.2 Condensed Nearest Neighbor Rule

Another under-sampling technique is the condensed nearest neighbor (CNN) rule [5], which is designed for the nearest neighbor decision rule (NN rule). For two bins called *store* and *grabbag*, the algorithm is defined as follows:

---

1. Put the whole sample of the minority class ($y = 1$) into *store*.
2. For $i = 1, \ldots, n_0$, repeat

   a. Predict class label of x_{0i} by NN using the sample in *store*.
   b. If x_{0i} is predicted correctly, then put it into *grabbag*, and otherwise, put it into *store*; here, $x_{01}, \ldots, x_{0n_0}$ are observations of the majority class ($y = 0$).

3. For the sample in *grabbag*, repeat step 2 until *grabbag* converges.
4. Output *store* as a consistent subset of the majority class.

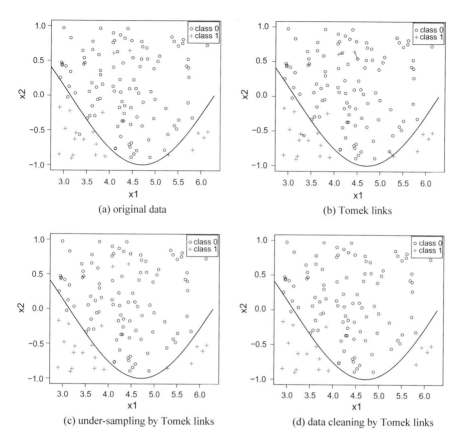

Fig. 1.1 Under-sampling by Tomek links

A consistent subset is a subset of the majority class that correctly predicts the class labels of the remaining observations of the majority class. The redundant observations for classification are removed by the CNN rule as shown in Fig. 1.2, in which the original data in (a) of Fig. 1.1 were under-sampled by CNN. Only observations of the majority class that is close to those of the minority class are preserved. The amount of reduction is relatively large compared to the result obtained with Tomek links. There are two cases in which *grabbag* converges: one in which the number of observations in *grabbag* reaches zero, and another in which no observation in *grabbag* is transferred to *store*. Note that in this algorithm, the number of observations in *store* monotonically increases.

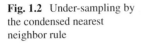

Fig. 1.2 Under-sampling by
the condensed nearest
neighbor rule

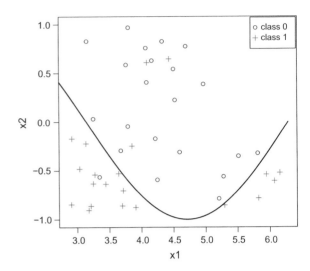

1.1.2   Over-Sampling Techniques

1.1.2.1   Synthetic Minority Over-Sampling Technique (SMOTE)

In SMOTE, observations of the minority class are over-sampled without duplications
based on k-nearest neighbors of the minority class. This approach originated from
the field of handwritten character recognition.

For $i = 1, \ldots, n_1$, repeat the following steps:

1. Compute k-nearest neighbors for the ith observation of the minority class
2. Choose one observation from the k-nearest neighbors, and denote it as x_{1j} ($j \neq i$).
3. Compute the difference $dif = x_{1j} - x_{1i}$.
4. Sample a random variable u from the standard uniform distribution U([0, 1]).
5. Generate the synthetic observation $x_{1i}^* = x_{1i} + u * dif$.

This algorithm results in 100% over-sampling (i.e., the sample size of the minority
class doubles). If less than 100% over-sampling is desired, then some portion of the
minority class is picked before the algorithm is processed. On the other hand, if
more than 100% over-sampling is desired, the user simply repeats the steps in the
algorithm more than n_1 times.

Table 1.1 Confusion matrix

Predicted class	True class		
	$y = 0$	$y = 1$	Total
$\hat{y} = 0$ (negative)	a	b	$a + b$
$\hat{y} = 1$ (positive)	c	d	$c + d$
Total	$n_0 (= a + c)$	$n_1 (= b + d)$	n

1.1.2.2 Borderline SMOTE

This method focuses on the minority class ($y = 1$) around the borderline between observations of $y = 0$ and $y = 1$ [4]. First, we conduct k-nearest neighbor analysis for the minority observations $x_{11}, \ldots, x_{1n_1}$ using the whole data set. We denote k' as the number of majority observations among the k-nearest neighbors. Then we consider three types of classes for the minority observation x_{1j} ($j = 1, \ldots, n_1$):

- x_{1j} is categorized as *noise* when $k = k'$. That is, x_{1j} is totally surrounded by majority observations
- x_{1j} is categorized as *danger* when $k/2 \leq k' < k$, which is likely to be near the borderline.
- x_{1j} is categorized as *safe* when $0 \leq k' < k/2$, which is likely far from the borderline.

Then, for the observations belonging to *danger*, SMOTE is conducted to increase the sample size of the minority class.

1.2 Evaluation Measures

It is also difficult to evaluate classification performance on imbalanced data. This is clearly demonstrated by a confusion matrix or an error matrix, in which each row represents predicted classes ($\hat{y} = 0$, $\hat{y} = 1$) and each column represents the true classes ($y = 0$, $y = 1$), as shown in Table 1.1. Each element shows the number of observations assigned according to the true and predicted classes. Several measures are derived from the confusion matrices as follows [10]:

- Accuracy is the proportion of observations that are correctly classified. That is,

$$\text{Accuracy} = \frac{a + d}{n}.$$

- Recall or Sensitivity or true positive rate (TPR) is the proportion of the observations of class $y = 1$ that are correctly predicted or classified as positives ($\hat{y} = 1$). That is,

$$\text{Recall} = \frac{d}{b+d} = \frac{d}{n_1},$$

where n_1 is the number of observations of class $y = 1$.

- Inverse Recall or Specificity or true negative rate (TNR) is the proportion of observations of class $y = 0$ that are correctly predicted or classified as negatives ($\hat{y} = 0$). That is,

$$\text{Inverse Recall} = \frac{a}{a+c} = \frac{a}{n_0},$$

where n_0 is the number of observations of class $y = 0$.

- Positive Predictive Value or Precision is the proportion of predicted positives that are truly positives. That is,

$$\text{Precision} = \frac{d}{c+d}.$$

- Negative Predictive Value is the counterpart of Positive Predictive Value. That is,

$$\text{Negative Predictive Value} = \frac{a}{a+b}.$$

- F-measure is the harmonic mean of Recall and Precision:

$$\begin{aligned}
\text{F-measure} &= \frac{2}{\frac{1}{\text{Recall}} + \frac{1}{\text{Precision}}} \\
&= \frac{2 \times \text{Recall} \times \text{Precision}}{\text{Recall} + \text{Precision}} \\
&= \frac{2d}{b+c+2d}.
\end{aligned}$$

The large value of F-measure means that both Recall and Precision are large.

- G-mean is the geometric mean of Recall and Inverse Recall:

$$\begin{aligned}
\text{G-mean} &= \sqrt{\text{Recall} \times \text{Inverse Recall}} \\
&= \sqrt{\frac{ad}{(b+d)(a+c)}}.
\end{aligned}$$

- AUC is the area under the ROC curve [13], which is a plot of ($1 -$ Inverse Recall, Recall) or (False Positive Rate, True Positive Rate) when a threshold moves in $(-\infty, \infty)$. This measure is insensitive to imbalance of the class labels of the data sets, which is investigated in detail in the subsequent section.

Note that all measures above have values between 0 and 1. We will now examine the sensitivity of these measures to imbalance of sample sizes of the class labels. Suppose $x_0 \sim N(0, I)$ and $x_1 \sim N(\mu_1, I)$, where $\mu_1 = (1, 1)^\top$. In the scatter plot in Fig. 1.3, the sample sizes of $y = 0$ and $y = 1$ are 100 and 10 in the left panel

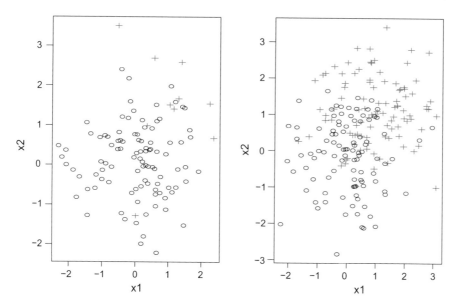

Fig. 1.3 Scatter plots of imbalanced data (left panel) and balanced data (right panel)

(imbalanced case), and 100 and 100 in the right panel (balanced case). The random variables are generated 100 times, and the evaluation measures are plotted based on Fisher's linear discriminant analysis as shown in Fig. 1.4. As seen in the boxplots, there are large gaps between the imbalanced and balanced cases except for the values of AUC. Moreover, the variances of Recall, Precision, F-measure, and G-mean are larger in the imbalanced case than in the balanced case. The values of accuracy in the imbalanced case are ostensibly improved because almost all observations, in which very few positives are present, are predicted to be negatives. Hence, we have to take extreme care of evaluation measures when we deal with imbalanced data sets.

1.2.1 Area Under the Receiver Operating Characteristic Curve

The area under the ROC has the advantage that it is not affected by an imbalance in sample size; hence, it can evaluate classification accuracy appropriately even if we deal with imbalanced data sets. It consists of a true positive rate (TPR) and a false positive rate (FPR) as follows.

For the discriminant function $F(x)$ and a threshold value c, FPR and TPR are defined as

$$\text{FPR}(c) = \int_{F(x)>c} g_0(x)dx, \ \text{TPR}(c) = \int_{F(x)>c} g_1(x)dx$$

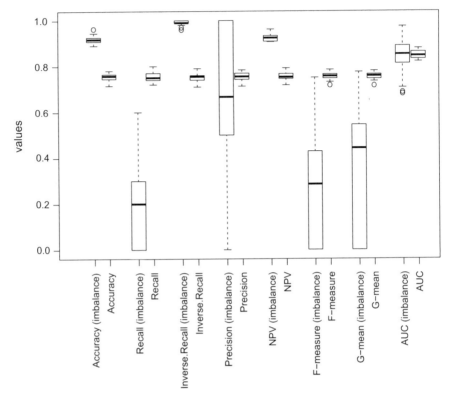

Fig. 1.4 Boxplot of several measures based on Fisher's linear discriminant analysis using balanced and imbalanced data generated by normal distributions

as illustrated in Fig. 1.5. These quantities are independent of the prior probabilities $P(y = 0)$ and $P(y = 1)$; hence, they are insensitive to the imbalance of sample sizes in $y = 0$ and $y = 1$. The ROC curve is a trajectory of these quantities, and is defined as

$$\text{ROC}(F) = \{(\text{FPR}(c), \text{TPR}(c)) | c \in \mathbb{R}\}.$$

Accordingly, the area under the ROC curve (AUC) is defined as

$$\text{AUC}(F) = \int_{-\infty}^{\infty} \text{TPR}(c) d\text{FPR}(c)$$

$$= \int \int \text{H}(F(x_1) - F(x_0)) g_0(x_0) g_1(x_1) dx_0 dx_1,$$

where $\text{H}(\cdot)$ is the Heaviside function: $\text{H}(z) = 1$ if $z \geq 0$ and 0 otherwise [1]. Empirically, it is expressed as

Fig. 1.5 Illustration of the false positive rate and the true positive rate based on a threshold c for probability density functions of $y = 0$ and $y = 1$

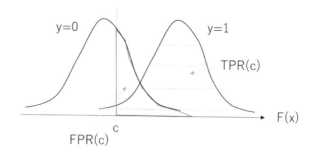

$$\overline{\text{AUC}}(F) = \frac{1}{n_0 n_2} \sum_{i=1}^{n_0} \sum_{j=1}^{n_1} \text{H}(F(x_{1j}) - F(x_{0i})),$$

where $\{x_{01}, \ldots, x_{0n_0}\}$ and $\{x_{11}, \ldots, x_{0n_1}\}$ are samples of $y = 0$ and $y = 1$, respectively. The statistical properties of the approximated empirical AUC have also been investigated in the framework of machine learning [6, 7].

1.2.2 Optimality of Evaluation Measures

The evaluation measures are upper bounded, so their optimal values depend on the discriminant function $F(x)$. For a threshold value c, the optimal values of FPR(c) and TPR(c) are attained by the density ratio $g_1(x)/g_0(x)$, where $g_0(x)$ and $g_1(x)$ are probability density functions of $y = 0$ and $y = 1$ [3, 7, 8]. Hence, we have

$$F_{\text{opt}} = \underset{F}{\text{argmax}} \ \text{AUC}(F),$$

where $F_{\text{opt}}(x) = g_1(x)/g_0(x)$. Similarly, the Positive Predictive Value (PPV, also called Precision), and negative predictive value (NPV) are maximized by F_{opt} because they are expressed as

$$\text{PPV}(c) = \frac{\text{TPR}(c) \times P(y = 1)}{\text{TPR}(c) \times P(y = 1) + \text{FPR}(c) \times P(y = 0)}$$

$$\text{NPV}(c) = \frac{(1 - \text{FPR}(c)) \times P(y = 0)}{(1 - \text{FPR}(c))P(y = 0) + (1 - \text{TPR}(c)) \times P(y = 1)}.$$

F-measure and G-mean are expressed as

$$\text{F-measure}(c) = \frac{2}{1/\text{TPR}(c) + 1/\text{PPV}(c)}$$

$$\text{G-mean}(c) = \sqrt{\text{TPR}(c) \times (1 - \text{FPR}(c))},$$

so they are also maximized by F_{opt}. Hence, the purpose of this classification is to estimate the density ratio $g_1(x)/g_0(x)$ with great accuracy using sophisticated statistical methods.

References

1. Bamber D (1975) The area above the ordinal dominance graph and the area below the receiver operating characteristic graph. J Math Psychol 12:387–415
2. Chawla NV (2010) Data mining for imbalanced datasets: an overview. Springer, MA, pp 875–886
3. Eguchi S, Copas J (2002) A class of logistic-type discriminant functions. Biometrika 89:1–22
4. Han H, Wang WY, Mao BH (2005) Borderline-SMOTE: a new over-sampling method in imbalanced data sets learning. In: Advances in intelligent computing, pp 878–887
5. Hart PE (1968) The condensed nearest neighbor rule. IEEE Trans Inf Theory 14:515–516
6. Komori O (2011) A boosting method for maximization of the area under the ROC curve. Ann Inst Stat Math 63:961–979
7. Komori O, Eguchi S (2010) A boosting method for maximizing the partial area under the ROC curve. BMC Bioinform 11:314
8. McIntosh MW, Pepe MS (2002) Combining several screening tests: optimality of the risk score. Biometrics 58:657–664
9. Nguyen HM, Coopery EW, Kamei K (2011) Borderline over-sampling for imbalanced data classification. Int J Knowl Eng Soft Data Parad 3:4–21
10. Powers DMW (2011) Evaluation: from precision, recall and F-measure to ROC, informedness, markedness and correlation. J Mach Learn Technol 2:37–63
11. Prati RC, Batista GE, Monard MC (2009) Data mining with imbalanced class distributions: concepts and methods. In: Indian international conference artificial intelligence, pp 359–376
12. Tomek I (1976) Two modifications of CNN. IEEE Trans Syst Man Cybern 6:769–772
13. Zhou X, Obuchowski NA, McClish DK (2002) Statistical methods in diagnostic medicine. Wiley, New York

Chapter 2
Weighted Logistic Regression

Abstract We consider an asymmetric logistic regression model as an example of a weighted logistic regression model, where the weights in the estimating equation vary according to the explanatory variables, thereby alleviating the imbalance of effective sample sizes between class labels $y = 0$ and $y = 1$. This model is extended to have a double robust property based on a propensity score, so that it has consistent estimators. We illustrate the utility of both models using the RAM and FAO data from fishery science.

Keywords Asymmetric logistic regression · Double robust · Fishery science · Propensity score

2.1 RAM Legacy Database

The disproportional relation between global fishing efforts and fish stocks in the oceans, described as "too many fishers chasing too few fish," causes massive economic and biological losses [2], depriving of their livelihoods millions of people who depend on fisheries [18]. A typical example is the collapse of the northern cod population off Newfoundland in 1993 [34] due to the poor recruitment of cod to the fishery. In this context, a great deal of attention has been paid to estimation of the status of fisheries worldwide. One approach is to use trends of time series of catch data, in which we assume that the amount of catch increases in the early stage of fishing and subsequently declines due to overexploitation [36]. We then compare the current value of catch with the highest value ever recorded. This is generally called the catch-based method [18], and it is widely employed because the data is easily obtained and publicly available from the Food and Agriculture Organization (FAO). However, catches vary due to several external factors such as the hour of fishing, gear technology, unreported fishing, regulations, subsidies to fisheries, and so on [2, 7]. Hence, a large catch does not always indicate an abundance of the stock, resulting in controversies over predictions about global fishery status in the middle of the twenty-first century [47] and a contentious debate about the utility of catch data in assessing stock status [38].

On the other hand, stock assessment data such as the RAM legacy database [40] provides us with intrinsic information about the abundance of stocks, such as biomass or exploitation rate, which are used to assess the conditions of large marine ecosystems [48]. It should be noted, however, that stock assessment has a limited sample size due to its financial cost, so it does not represent all stocks worldwide rather a subset of species included in research surveys and other fishery data [45, 48]. Recently, new methods have been proposed to incorporate globally available data such as catch, life history in FishBase [17] and information about the location of fishing, and stock assessment data in order to produce more reliable estimations of global stock status [11, 45]. First, the authors build a statistical model to connect the abundance and the fishery-related data using limited amounts of assessed stock data, and then apply the results to the large amount of unassessed data in the FAO database in order to derive global collapse probabilities or relative biomass values. In particular, [45] considered a mixed-effect logistic regression model, which is widely used in ecology [49], to allow for unexpected region-dependent variations. However, they faced difficulty in estimating the collapse probabilities because of the highly imbalanced sample size (7766 non-collapsed stocks vs. 431 collapsed stocks overall, observed from 1950 to 2008 in the RAM legacy database); especially, the probability of correctly classifying the collapsed stocks to be collapsed (true positive rate) is especially poorly estimated. Moreover, the values of biomass in the observation years and at maximum sustainable yield (MSY), which determine the status of collapsed versus non-collapsed, are in fact estimated from biomass dynamics models, resulting in uncertainty about the stock status.

To deal with the imbalanced nature of the sample size and the uncertainty about the definition of stock status, we propose an asymmetric logistic regression model based on the idea of a contamination model [9], in which an additional parameter, κ, is introduced. In this model, we assume that some of the observations about collapsed stocks are distributed in the same way as those of non-collapsed stocks. By observing the estimation equation or the score function, we find that more weight is placed on observations of collapsed stocks, thereby alleviating the effects of imbalanced sample size. We note that our proposed method can be easily implemented via a small modification of a logit link function in the generalized linear model. In addition, we can incorporate the mixed effects into our proposed model easily. For example, it is sufficient to modify the user-defined link function in lme4 package [4] in the R statistical software.

2.2 Asymmetric Logistic Regression

We developed an asymmetric logistic regression with mixed effects to construct a model for predicting fishery status based on stock assessments in the RAM data [40]. In this approach, we use an asymmetric logistic function as a link function in the generalized linear mixed model to allow for the imbalance in sample size and uncertainty of class labeling (collapsed vs. non-collapsed). As seen in Fig. 2.1,

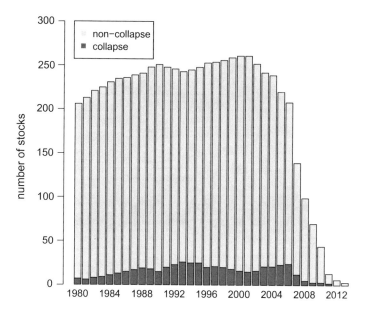

Fig. 2.1 Bar plots of number of stocks in RAM data from 1980 to 2013, where the red and gray bars indicate the numbers of collapsed and non-collapsed stocks, respectively

there are very few collapsed stocks and a great many non-collapsed stocks in the RAM data. In such cases, the typical statistical methods such as logistic regression models do not work properly: predictions for non-collapsed stocks are relatively accurate, but the predictions for collapsed stocks are rather inaccurate due to the small sample size. Consequently, the estimated collapse probabilities for collapsed stocks are underestimated, resulting in a large value of undetected error probabilities for stocks that are actually at risk of collapsing.

Our aim is to propose a robust method for predicting stock status in such irregular situations. Let $y \in \{0, 1\}$ be a class label for non-collapsed ($y = 0$) and collapsed ($y = 1$), and let x and z be explanatory variables associated with fixed and random effects, respectively. Then, the conditional probability of y given (x, z, b) in a mixed-effect asymmetric logistic regression is formulated with a nonnegative parameter κ as

$$P_\kappa(y = 1 | x, z; \eta) = \frac{\exp\{\eta(x, z)\} + \kappa}{1 + \exp\{\eta(x, z)\} + \kappa}, \tag{2.1}$$

where η is called a predictor and has a form like $\eta(x, z) = \alpha + \beta^\top x + b^\top z$, α is an intercept, and β and b are fixed and random effects, respectively. Note that if $\kappa = 0$, then it reduces to a conditional probability in the usual logistic regression.

$$P_0(y = 1|x, z; \eta) = \frac{\exp\{\eta(x, z)\}}{1 + \exp\{\eta(x, z)\}}. \tag{2.2}$$

Let $f(x, z|y)$ be a conditional probability density function of (x, z) given y. Then by Bayes theorem, the logistic regression model is written as

$$P_0(y = 1|x, z; \eta_0) = \frac{\pi_1 f(x, z|y = 1)}{\pi_0 f(x, z|y = 0) + \pi_1 f(x, z|y = 1)}, \tag{2.3}$$

where

$$\eta_0(x, z) = \log \frac{\pi_1 f(x, z|y = 1)}{\pi_0 f(x, z|y = 0)}, \tag{2.4}$$

and $P(y = 0) = \pi_0$ and $P(y = 1) = \pi_1$. Similarly, if we assume that the true conditional probability function of (x, z) given $y = 1$ is contaminated with a mixing proportion δ $(0 \le \delta < 1)$ as

$$f^*(x, z|y = 1) = (1 - \delta)f(x, z|y = 1) + \delta f(x, z|y = 0), \tag{2.5}$$

then we have

$$P_{\gamma\delta}(y = 1|x, z; \eta_1) = \frac{\pi_1 f^*(x, z|y = 1)}{\pi_0 f(x, z|y = 0) + \pi_1 f^*(x, z|y = 1)}, \tag{2.6}$$

where

$$\eta_1(x, z) = \eta_0(x, z) + \log(1 - \delta), \tag{2.7}$$

and $\gamma = \pi_1/\pi_0$. Hence, in the asymmetric logistic regression model in (2.1), we assume $\eta_1(x, z)$ has a linear form like $\alpha + \beta^\top x + b^\top z$. Model in (2.5) is referred to as a contaminated model [9, 20, 44]. The value of δ indicates how much the conditional probability of x given $y = 1$ is contaminated by the conditional probability of x given $y = 0$, and the estimation of δ can be performed by estimation of κ in (2.1) using a relation such as $\delta = \kappa/\gamma$. Note that $P_\kappa(y = 1|x, z; \eta) = \pi_1$ if $f(y = 1|x, z) = f(y = 0|x, z)$, which is the same property satisfied in the usual logistic regression model in (2.3). Such modeling is useful when the information of class label $y = 1$ is not well-specified but that of $y = 0$ is presumably well-specified by the usual logistic model in practical situations. This is the case in the RAM data analysis as shown in the subsequent discussion.

Weighted Logistic Regression

The estimating equations of the asymmetric logistic regression model [25] regarding to β and b are expressed as

$$\sum_{i=1}^{n} w(\eta_i)\left\{y_i - P_\kappa(y_i = 1|x_i, z_i; \eta)\right\}x_i = 0 \tag{2.8}$$

and

$$\sum_{i=1}^{n} w(\eta_i)\left\{y_i - P_\kappa(y_i = 1|x_i, z_i; \eta)\right\}z_i = D^{-1}b, \tag{2.9}$$

where $w(\eta_i) = \exp(\eta_i)/\{\exp(\eta_i) + \kappa\}$, $\eta_i = \alpha + \beta^\top x_i + b^\top z_i$ and $b \sim N(0, D)$. These are derived from the integrated likelihood function for mixed-effects model in a manner similar to that described in [6]. A large value of η_i means that the weight $w(\eta_i)$ is almost equal to 1, which is the case for positive observations whose sample size is very low in imbalanced data sets. On the other hand, the small value of η_i means that $w(\eta_i)$ is almost equal to 0, which is the case for negative observations whose sample size is relatively large. Hence, the weight function plays a role in alleviating imbalance in sample size, and the value of weight can be estimated by information criteria such as AIC [1] or BIC [43].

In the original weighted logistic regression model [28, 29, 31], the corresponding estimating equations are

$$\sum_{i=1}^{n} w_i\left\{y_i - P_0(y_i = 1|x_i, z_i; \eta)\right\}x_i = 0 \tag{2.10}$$

and

$$\sum_{i=1}^{n} w_i\left\{y_i - P_0(y_i = 1|x_i, z_i; \eta)\right\}z_i = D^{-1}b, \tag{2.11}$$

where $w_i = (\tau/\bar{y})y_i + (1 - \tau)/(1 - \bar{y})(1 - y_i)$ with τ being the prior probability $P(y = 1)$. In practice, τ is replaced with a value estimated based on prior knowledge of the population probability or acquired from previous surveys. However, it is often the case that τ is unknown and must be estimated by the data in analysis. Another interesting weight function is derived from the γ-divergence-based loss function [24]:

$$\sum_{i=1}^{n} w_\gamma(\eta_i)\left\{y_i - P_0(y_i = 1|x_i, z_i; \eta)\right\}x_i = 0 \tag{2.12}$$

and

$$\sum_{i=1}^{n} w_\gamma(\eta_i)\Big\{y_i - P_0(y_i = 1 | x_i, z_i; \eta)\Big\}z_i = D^{-1}b, \qquad (2.13)$$

where

$$w_\gamma(\eta_i) = \left[\frac{\exp\{y_i(1+\gamma)\eta_i\}}{1 + \exp\{(1+\gamma)\eta_i\}}\right]^{\frac{\gamma}{1+\gamma}},$$

where $\gamma > 0$. The clear difference between weight functions $w(\eta_i)$ and $w_\gamma(\eta_i)$ is that the latter depends on the class label y_i; whereas the former does not. For $w_\gamma(\eta_i)$, we observe that a large negative η_i with $y_i = 1$ or a large positive η_i with $y_i = 0$ reduces the value of the weight, decreasing the effects of observations that are likely to be mislabeled. Hence, $w_\gamma(\eta_i)$ does not alleviate the imbalance of sample sizes of $y = 0$ and $y = 1$ unlike the role of $w(\eta_i)$ in the asymmetric logistic regression model.

2.3 Data Description and Preprocessing

The most common and widely used global stock assessment dataset is available from the RAM Legacy Stock Assessment Database [40], which has 284 assessed stocks and time series catch data from 1950 to 2013. The latest dataset includes information from North-West Pacific (Asia) and Antarctic Ocean, regions for which abundant data was not available in the past. Although the database does not fully cover all fishing areas worldwide, and biased toward commercially important species in developed nations [23], it is still essential for the estimation of global fishery status [11, 45, 48]. The dataset mainly includes the amount of catch and the biomass B, and the biomass at maximum sustainable yield, B_{msy}. Stock status is determined to be collapsed or non-collapsed according to the value of B/B_{msy}. If B/B_{msy} is less than 0.2, the stock is assigned to be collapsed: otherwise, it is assigned to be non-collapsed, as in [11, 45, 48]. However, note that the values of biomass are estimated by several modeling techniques such as virtual population analysis, catch-at-age model, biomass dynamics model, integrated model, and others, depending on the amounts of information of each stock. Moreover, the precision of the estimated values varies depending on the methods used. Other fishery-related variables used in this analysis are trophic level (TL) and maximum recorded length of stock in life history (Lmax), which are available in FishBase [17]. Catch data with more than 1,000 tons accumulated during observation years was included in the analysis by analogy with [19, 45, 47]. To remove the drastic variability in the raw values of catch data [39], we applied a 3-year moving average filter to obtain smoothed catch values. Then, the relative catch (RC) is calculated such that the smoothed value is divided by the highest value ever recorded prior to the observation year [45]. The geographic region codes are also incorporated into the analysis to allow for region-dependent variability as well as International Standard Statistical Classification of Aquatic Animals and Plants (ISSCAAP), which is illustrated in Table 2.1. Because of the sparsity of the RAM data in terms of regions for which data is available, we summarized the region codes into five categories according to the number of assessed stocks: NW Atlantic (Region = 1), NE Atlantic (Region = 2), NE Pacific (Region = 3), SW Pacific (Region = 4), and other regions (Region = 5), which correspond to four data-rich regions and data-poor regions [45]. The information from ISSCAAP was also simplified into two categories, i.e., demersal fish (Group = 1) and non-demersal fish (Group = 0).

R Code

The RAM and FAO data from 1980 to 2013 are available in the DRAL package provided by [26], which is prepared as a.tar.gz format in the journal. It can be used as follows:

```
> install.packages("DRAL_1.0.tar.gz",type="source",repo=NULL)
> library(DRAL)
> help(ramfao)
> data(ramfao)
> dim(ramfao)
[1] 64984      10
> ramfao[1:5,]
        RC Lmax   TL Group Year Year2 Region   RB      Y Delta
8765 0.7272074   66 4.1     1   11   121      4 1.25 FALSE     1
8766 0.6196783   66 4.1     1   12   144      4 1.23 FALSE     1
8767 0.4843820   66 4.1     1   13   169      4 1.22 FALSE     1
8768 0.5511762   66 4.1     1   14   196      4 1.20 FALSE     1
8769 0.8268979   66 4.1     1   15   225      4 1.18 FALSE     1
```

The variable year starts from 1980 (Year = 0) and ends with 2013 (Year = 33). The indicator variable Δ (Delta) has a value 1 for stocks in the RAM data, and a value 0 for those in the FAO data. The standardized data is also available to stabilize the estimation procedure.

```
> data(ramfao.st)
```

We use the data in 1980 and apply an asymmetric logistic regression mixed-effects model with $\kappa = 0.01$ using glmer in the lmer4 package [4].

```
> library(lme4)
> kappa=0.01
> data=ramfao.st[ramfao$Year==0&ramfao$Delta==1,]
> result=glmer(Y~RC+TL+Lmax+(RC|Region),data=data,
                   family=binomial(link=link.eta(kappa)))
```

Table 2.1 The number of stocks in the RAM data categorized by region and ISSCAAP category

Region	ISSCAAP category												
	31	32	33	34	35	36	37	38	42	43	44	45	55
Antarctic	0	0	0	10	0	0	0	0	0	0	0	0	0
Atlantic Ocean	0	0	0	0	0	778	0	0	0	0	0	0	0
Australia	0	0	130	278(10)	0	0	0	0	0	0	0	0	0
Canada East Coast	116(15)	164(43)	0	46	0	0	0	0	0	0	0	0	22(3)
Canada West Coast	98	89	0	100	270(32)	0	0	0	0	0	0	0	0
Europe (non EU)	40(4)	380(2)	0	0	18	0	58(13)	0	0	0	0	0	0
European Union	273	408(33)	0	0	316(15)	0	32	0	0	0	0	0	0
Indian Ocean	0	0	0	0	0	285	0	0	0	0	0	0	0
Mediterranean/Black Sea	0	0	0	0	0	84	0	0	0	0	0	0	0
New Zealand	0	169	85	756	0	0	56	0	0	255(21)	0	0	0
Other	0	0	0	0	0	0	0	0	0	0	0	0	0
Pacific Ocean	0	0	0	0	0	608(10)	0	0	0	0	0	0	0
Russia & Japan	0	87	0	0	0	0	0	0	0	0	0	0	0
South Africa	0	128	0	76	40(3)	0	61	0	0	33	0	0	0
South America	0	60(7)	0	0	29	0	29	0	0	0	0	0	0
US Alaska	348(7)	167	75(44)	314	0	0	0	0	27	0	23	0	0
US East Coast	322(149)	200(66)	113(13)	166(22)	87(2)	0	102	0	0	24	0	21	29(20)
US Southeast/Gulf	0	0	199(22)	39	38	69(3)	16(5)	0	0	0	0	0	0
US West Coast	302	40	263(6)	1143(23)	0	44	59(5)	119	0	0	0	0	0

The number in parenthesis indicates the number of collapsed stocks. 31 = Founders halibuts, soles; 32 = Cods, hakes, haddocks; 33 = Redfishes, basses, congers (coastal); 34 = Jacks, mullets, sauries (demersal); 35 = Herrings, sardines anchovies; 36 = Tunas, bonitos, billfishes; 37 = Mackerels, snoeks, cutlassfishes (pelagic); 38 = Sharks, rays, chimeras; 42 = Sea spiders, crabs; 43 = Lobsters, spiny rock lobsters; 44 = Squat lobsters; 45 = Shrimps, prawns, winkles, conchs; 55 = Scallops, pectens

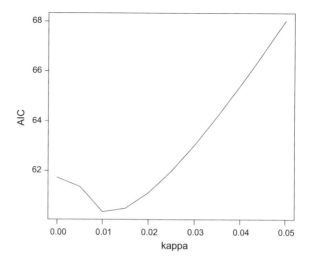

Fig. 2.2 Values of AIC based on the asymmetric logistic regression using RAM data from 1980

Actually, $\kappa = 0.01$ is optimal as shown in Fig. 2.2.
    Then we have the following result:

```
> result
Generalized linear mixed model fit by maximum likelihood
(Laplace Approximation) [glmerMod]
 Family: binomial   ( link.eta(0.01) )
Formula: Y ~ RC + TL + Lmax + (RC | Region)
   Data: data
     AIC      BIC   logLik deviance df.resid
 60.3507  83.8798 -23.1754  46.3507      206
Random effects:
 Groups Name         Std.Dev. Corr
 Region (Intercept) 1.803885
        RC          0.002363 0.98
Number of obs: 213, groups:  Region, 5
Fixed Effects:
(Intercept)            RC           TL          Lmax
     -7.095        -3.032       -2.970         1.393
convergence code 0; 1 optimizer warnings; 0 lme4 warnings
```

The values of AIC, BIC, and log-likelihood are obtained as well as the estimates of
random effects and fixed effects. The link function `link.eta` is defined as

```
link.eta=function(kappa){
  linkfun <- function(mu)log((1+kappa)*mu-kappa/(1-mu))
  linkinv <- function(eta)(kappa+exp(eta))/(1+exp(eta)+kappa)
  mu.eta <- function(eta)exp(eta)/(1+exp(eta)+kappa)^2
  valideta <- function(eta) TRUE
  link <- paste0("link.eta(", kappa, ")")
  structure(list(linkfun = linkfun, linkinv = linkinv,
```

```
                        mu.eta = mu.eta, valideta = valideta,
                        name = link), class = "link-glm")
    }
```

The inverse link function corresponds with the model of asymmetric logistic regression in (2.1).

2.4 Double Robust Asymmetric Logistic Regression Model

2.4.1 Selection Bias

In conservation ecology, predicting population abundance is one of the most important and fundamental applications of ecological and statistical models in practice [13]. The data used in such analysis is usually assumed to be representative of the underlying population. But it is often not the case due to the nonrandom selection of the data [14]. This problem is called selection bias, leading to biased and unreliable results in data analysis. This is common in ecology [8, 16, 27] as well as epidemiology and medicine [12, 21].

In fisheries, the selection bias is recognized in the framework of meta-analysis [22], in which it is suggested that fish stocks in an available database could be selected non-randomly for several reasons such as economic interest and differences in whether they were assessed by developed or developing nations. Together, these biases can result in overestimation of productivity or underestimation of depensation of the target population. To tackle this problem, they suggest the idea of the propensity score [41], which is widely used in clinical studies and quantifies the extent to which the sampled data is biased. The propensity score was recently incorporated into the assessment of biological effects of catch share fisheries [10, 32] and introduced in guidelines for fishery data analysis [46].

2.4.2 Difference Between RAM and FAO Data

To date, very little attention has been paid to selection bias in predictions of fish stock abundance. The fundamental and naive approach is to compare the current catch value with the highest one recorded in the past. Then, the fish stock is estimated as collapsed or non-collapsed according to the ratio of the two values with a threshold; this is called as the catch-based method [19]. Worldwide stock status estimation has yielded the shocking prediction that all fish stocks will be collapsed by the middle of the twenty-first century [47], which is based on an assumption that catch will tend to reflect abundance [37]. The criticism is that catch data, which is generally obtained from FAO database [15], does not accurately indicate the abundance of fish stocks because the catch values are easily affected by the hour of fishing, gear technology, unreported fishing, regulations, and subsidies to fisheries [2, 7]. Also, the effect of recovered fish stocks is neglected in the analysis above, leading to an incorrect projection of the fish stock abundance [5].

On the other hand, the stock assessment database [33] has played an essential role in estimating stock abundance because it integrates not only time series of catch data but also other biological information such as growth, maturation, natural mortality rates, and catch-per-unit-of-effort, in order to obtain the more reliable criteria such as biomass and exploitation rate [40]. This database is called the RAM legacy stock assessment database (RAM data), which is already introduced in Sect. 2.1, in honor of the late Ransom A. Myers who was a world-renowned fisheries conservation biologist [35]. Biological reference points such as biomass and exploitation rates are essential for sustainable fishery management [30].

2.4.3 Propensity Score

The clear difference between the RAM and the FAO data is that biomass, which is used for determining collapsed versus non-collapsed, is available in the RAM data but missing from the FAO data. Moreover, the RAM data suffers from high selection bias such as temporal, geographic, and taxonomic biases [40]. Some stocks may be more or less likely to enter the RAM data depending on their commercial benefits or the management of the regional fishery agencies to which they belong. To allow for the fact that biomass data is missing as well as the non-randomness of the selection, the propensity score [41], which is widely used in medical or clinical studies, can also be employed in fishery science [46]. Here, the propensity score is a probability that a stock will be present in the RAM data, which can be modeled as

$$P(\Delta = 1|x_i) = \frac{\exp(\alpha^\top x_i)}{1 + \kappa \exp(\alpha^\top x_i)}, \quad i = 1, \ldots, n, \qquad (2.14)$$

where $\Delta_i = 1$ indicates that the stock i belongs to RAM data; $\Delta_i = 0$ indicates that it belongs to FAO data, and n is the total sample size of RAM and FAO data. Here, x_i is the ith p-dimensional variable, including both fixed and random effects, used for prediction; α is the corresponding coefficient, and κ (≥ 1) is a parameter that measures the extent to which the FAO data is heterogeneous in terms of the probability distribution in the asymmetric logistic regression. Note that this model reduces to the usual logistic regression model when $\kappa = 1$.

2.4.4 Model Formulation

In the preceding studies [11, 25, 45], the prediction models for abundance of marine stocks (collapse probability in our case) have been constructed using *only* RAM data, which is likely to suffer from high selection bias. This means that the information about the FAO data, which is globally collected and can be regarded as better reflecting global stock abundance, is not properly taken into account in the construction of prediction models, resulting in a biased estimation of abundance. To address this problem, we employ the double robust estimation for collapse probability based on the propensity score. Here "double robust" means that the model can do the estimation consistently (without bias) when either the model for the propensity score (missing data model) or the model for the prediction of collapse probability (outcome regression model) is correctly specified. Due to the frequency and near inevitability of model mis-specification, the property of double robustness is highly desirable [3]. Our proposed prediction model for collapsed ($y = 1$) or non-collapsed ($y = 0$) based on the variables x is formulated as

$$P(y = 1|x) = \frac{\left\{\exp(\beta^\top x) + \lambda\right\}\exp\{\phi\pi_\kappa(x;\alpha)^{-1}\}}{1 + \left\{\exp(\beta^\top x) + \lambda\right\}\exp\{\phi\pi_\kappa(x;\alpha)^{-1}\}}, \quad \lambda \geq 0 \quad (2.15)$$

where $\pi_\kappa(x;\alpha)$ denotes the propensity score in (2.14), i.e., $\pi_\kappa(x;\alpha) = \exp(\alpha^\top x)/\{1 + \kappa \exp(\alpha^\top x)\}$. When the parameter $\phi = 0$, then it becomes the asymmetric logistic regression model (AL) in [25]. When the parameter $\lambda = 0$, then it becomes the double robust logistic regression model (DRL) in [3, 42]. Hence, we call the model in (2.15) a double robust asymmetric logistic regression model (DRAL), which incorporates a property of AL that allows for asymmetry in probability distribution of the data, and a property of DRL that enables unbiased estimation based on the propensity score.

The estimation of the propensity score $P(\Delta = 1|x)$ and the collapse probability $P(y = 1|x)$ based on DRAL are implemented in the DRAL package.

```
> library(lme4)
> data(ramfao.st)
> estPS(Delta~Lmax+TL+RC+Group+(Group|Region),
            data=ramfao.st, grid.kappa=1+0:10/10)
```

where the optimal value of κ is determined by the grid search. It returns the optimal κ as 1.5; the AIC turns out to be 36200. The estimated linear predictor $\hat{\alpha}^\top x_i$ is

$$-2.33 + 0.076 \ RC_i + 0.36Lmax_i + 0.37TL_i + 2.38Group_i$$
$$+ \sum_{a \in \mathscr{F}} \hat{\alpha}_{r0} I(Region_i = a) + \sum_{a \in \mathscr{F}} \hat{\alpha}_{r1} I(Region_i = a)Group_i,$$

where the values are recorded as the PS.hat object. Then, based on the value of PS.hat, the collapse probability by DRAL is implemented as

```
> estDRAL(Y~Lmax+Group+Year2+RC+Year+(RC|Region),
            data=ramfao.st, grid.lambda=seq(0,10,by=2)/1000,PS=PS.hat)
```

This produces the linear predictor $\hat{\beta}^{\top} x_i$ as

$$-9.31 - 3.90 \ \text{RC}_i + 1.12\text{Lmax}_i + 0.47\text{Group}_i + 0.54\text{Year}_i - 0.75\text{Year}_i^2 \quad (2.16)$$
$$+ \sum_{a \in \mathscr{F}} \hat{\beta}_{r0} I\,(\text{Region}_i = a) + \sum_{a \in \mathscr{F}} \hat{\beta}_{r1} I\,(\text{Region}_i = a)\text{RC}_i,$$

where $\hat{\phi} = 0.046$. Here, we used the variables in the model which were selected using AIC. RC and Year^2 have negative impacts on the collapse probability; while, Lmax, Group, and Year have the positive impacts. See [26] for the more details of the estimation results.

References

1. Akaike H (1973) Information theory and an extension of the maximum likelihood principle. In: Second international symposium on information theory, pp 267–281
2. Arnason R, Kelleher K, Willmann R (2009) The sunken billions: the economic justification for fisheries reform. The World Bank, Washington
3. Bang H, Robins JM (2005) Doubly robust estimation in missing data and causal inference models. Biometrics 61:962–972
4. Bates D, Machler M, Bolker B, Walker S (2015) Fitting linear mixed-effects models using lme4
5. Branch TA (2008) Not all fisheries will be collapsed in 2048. Mar Policy 32:38–39
6. Breslow NE, Clayton DG (1993) Approximate inference in generalized linear mixed models. J Am Stat Assoc 88:9–25
7. Carruthers TR, Walters CJ, McAllister MK (2012) Evaluating methods that classify fisheries stock status using only fisheries catch data. Fish Res 119:66–79
8. Conn PB, Johnson DS, London J, Boveng PL (2012) Accounting for missing data when assessing availability in animal population surveys: an application to ice-associated seals in the Bering Sea. Methods Ecol Evol 3:1039–1046
9. Copas J (1988) Binary regression models for contaminated data. J R Stat Soc: Ser B 50:225–265
10. Costello C, Gaines SD, Lynham J (2008) Can catch shares prevent fisheries collapse? Science 321:1678–1681
11. Costello C, Ovando D, Hilborn R, Gaines SD, Deschenes O, Lester SE (2012) Status and solutions for the world's unassessed fisheries. Science 338:517–520
12. Ellenberg JH (1994) Selection bias in observational and experimental studies. Stat Med 13:557–567
13. Ferguson JM, Ponciano JM (2014) Predicting the process of extinction in experimental microcosms and accounting for interspecific interactions in single-species time series. Ecol Lett 17:251–259
14. Fieberg JR, Con PB (2014) A hidden Markov model to identify and adjust for selection bias: an example involving mixed migration strategies. Ecol Evol 4:1903–1912
15. Food and Agriculture Organization of the United Nations (1999) Food and Agricultural Organization International Plan of Action for the conservation and management of sharks (IPOA); 1999. ftp://ftp.fao.org/docrep/fao/006/x3170e/X3170E00.pdf
16. Frair JL, Fieberg J, Hebblewhite M, Cagnacci F, DeCesare NJ, Pedrotti L (2010) Resolving issues of imprecise and habitat-biased locations in ecological analyses using GPS telemetry data. Phil Trans R Soc B 365:2187–2200
17. Froese R, Pauly D (2014) FishBase. World Wide Web electronic publication www.fishbase.org

18. Froese R, Kesner-Reyes K (2002) Impact of fishing on the abundance of marine species. ICES CM 12:1–12
19. Froese R, Zeller D, Kleisner K, Pauly D (2012) What catch data can tell us about the status of global fisheries. Mar Biol 159:1283–1292
20. Hayashi K (2012) A boosting method with asymmetric mislabeling probabilities which depend on covariates. Comput Stat 27:203–218
21. Hernán MA, Hernández-Díaz S, Robins JM (2004) Epidemiology 15:615–625
22. Hilborn R, Liermann M (1998) Standing on the shoulders of giants: learning from experience in fisheries. Rev Fish Biol Fish 8:273–283
23. Hilborn R, Ovando D (2014) Reflections on the success of traditional fisheries management. ICES J Mar Sci. https://doi.org/10.1093/icesjms/fsu034
24. Hung H, Jou ZY, Huang SY (2018) Robust mislabel logistic regression without modeling mislabel probabilities. Biometrics 74:145–154
25. Komori O, Eguchi S, Ikeda S, Okamura H, Ichinokawa M, Nakayama S (2016) An asymmetric logistic regression model for ecological data. Methods Ecol Evol 7:249–260
26. Komori O, Eguchi S, Saigusa Y, Okamura H, Ichinokawa M (2017) Robust bias correction model for estimation of global trend in marine populations. Ecosphere 8:1–9
27. Kramer-Schadt S, Niedballa J, Pilgrim JD, Schröder B, Lindenborn J, Reinfelder V, Stillfried M, Heckmann I, Scharf AK, Augeri DM, Cheyne SM, Hearn AJ, Ross J, Macdonald DW, Mathai J, James Eaton, Marshall Andrew J, G.S., Rustam, R., Bernard, H., Alfred, R., Samejima, H., J. W. Duckworth and C.B.W., Belant, J.L., Hofer1, H. & Wilting, A. (2013) The importance of correcting for sampling bias in MaxEnt species distribution models. Divers Distrib 19:1336–1379
28. Maalouf M, Siddiqi M (2014) Weighted logistic regression for large-scale imbalanced and rare events data. Knowl-Based Syst 59:142–148
29. Maalouf M, Trafalis TB (2011) Robust weighted kernel logistic regression in imbalanced and rare events data. Comput Stat Data Anal 55:168–183
30. Mace PM (1994) Relationships between common biological reference points used as thresholds and targets of fisheries management strategies. Can J Fish Aquat Sci 51:110–122
31. Manski CF, Lerman SR (1977) The estimation of choice probabilities from choice based samples. Econometrica 45:1977–1988
32. Melnychuk MC, Essington TE, Branch TA, Heppell SS, Jensen OP, Link JS, Martell SJD, Parma AM, Pope JG, Smith ADM (2012) Can catch share fisheries better track management targets? Fish Fish 13:267–290
33. Myers RA, Bridson J, Barrowman NJ (1995) Summary of worldwide spawner and recruitment data. Canadian technical report of fisheries and aquatic sciences. No. 2020, p 312
34. Myers RA, Hutchings JA, Barrowman NJ (1997) Why do fish stocks collapse? the example of cod in Atlantic Canada. Ecol Appl 7:91–106
35. Pauly D (2007a) Obituary: Ransom Aldrich Myers (1952–2007). Nature 447:160
36. Pauly D (2007b) The sea around us project: documenting and communicating global fisheries impacts on marine ecosystems. J Hum Environ 36:290–295
37. Pauly D, Christensen V, Dalsgaard J, Froese R, Jr., FT (1998) How Pervasive is "Fishing downmarine food webs"? Science 282:1839
38. Pauly D, Hilborn R, Branch TA (2013) Fisheries: does catch reflect abundance? Nature 494:303–306
39. Pinsky ML, Jensen OP, Ricardc D, Palumbi SR (2011) Unexpected patterns of fisheries collapse in the world's oceans. Proc Natl Acad Sci U S A 108:8317–8322
40. Ricard D, Minto C, Jensen OP, Baum JK (2012) Examining the knowledge base and status of commercially exploited marine species with the RAM legacy stock assessment database. Fish Fish 13:380–398
41. Rosenbaum PR, Rubin DB (1983) The central role of the propensity score in observational studies for causal effects. Biometrics 70:41–55
42. Scharfstein DO, Rotnitzky A, Robins JM (1999) Adjusting for nonignorable drop-out using semiparametric nonresponse models. J Am Stat Assoc 94:1096–1120 (with Rejoinder, 1135–1146)

43. Schwarz G (1978) Estimating the dimension of a model. Ann Stat 6:461–464
44. Takenouchi T, Eguchi S (2004) Robustifying AdaBoost by adding the naive error rate. Neural Comput 16:767–787
45. Thorson JT, Branch TA, Jensen OP (2012) Using model-based inference to evaluate global fisheries status from landings, location, and life history data. Can J Fish Aquat Sci 69:645–655
46. Thorson JT, Cope JM, Kleisner KM, Samhouri JF, Shelton AO, Ward EJ (2015) Giants' shoulders 15 years later: lessons, challenges and guidelines in fisheries meta-analysis. Fish Fish 16:342–361
47. Worm B, Barbier EB, Beaumont N, Duffy JE, Folke C, Halpern BS, Jackson JBC, Lotze HK, Micheli F, Palumbi SR, Sala E, Selkoe KA, Stachowicz JJ, Watson R (2006) Impacts of biodiversity loss on ocean ecosystem services. Science 314:787–790
48. Worm B, Hilborn R, Baum JK, Branch TA, Collie JS, Costello C, Fogarty MJ, Fulton EA, Hutchings JA, Jennings S, Jensen OP, Lotze HK, Mace PM, McClanahan TR, Minto C, Palumbi SR, Parma AM, Ricard D, Rosenberg AA, Watson R, Zeller D (2009) Rebuilding global fisheries. Science 325:578–585
49. Zuur A, Ieno EN, Walker N, Saveliev AA, Smith GM (2009) Mixed effects models and extensions in ecology with R. Springer, New York

Chapter 3
β-Maxent

Abstract Maxent is very popular for estimating species distributions using environmental variables such as temperature, precipitation, elevation, and soil cat- egory, all of which are closely related to the habitat of the species of interest. It is designed for estimating a probability distribution that has maximum entropy subject to the condition that the sample means of environmental variables are equal to the population means. Maxent can deal with presence-only data, for which the records of positions of the species are available but those of absence of the species are not available. Hence, this kind of data can be regarded as the extreme case of imbalance data, where observations belonging to one class ($y = 0$ or $y = 1$) are totally miss- ing. We investigate the Maxent from the viewpoint of divergence and extend it by introducing β-divergence, a variant of the more general class of U-divergence.

Keywords Habitat distribution · Maxent · Presence-only data · U-divergence

3.1 U-Divergence

U-divergence, a special case of the Bregman divergence [8], is defined by a convex and strictly increasing function U. It measures the closeness between two probability functions $\pi(x)$ and $\pi'(x)$, which are defined in a sample space $\mathscr{X}$.

$$D_U(\pi, \pi') = - \sum_{x \in \mathscr{X}} \pi(x) \left\{ \xi(\pi'(x)) - \xi(\pi(x)) \right\} + \sum_{x \in \mathscr{X}} U(\xi(\pi'(x))) - U(\xi(\pi(x))),$$

where u is the derivative of U, ξ is the inverse of u. If we consider a distance function $d(\cdot, \cdot)$, we have

$$D_U(\pi, \pi') = \sum_{x \in \mathscr{X}} d(\xi(\pi(x)), \xi(\pi'(x))),$$

O. Komori and S. Eguchi, *Statistical Methods for Imbalanced Data in Ecological and Biological Studies*, JSS Research Series in Statistics,
https://doi.org/10.1007/978-4-431-55570-4_3

where

$$d(s, t) = U(t) - U(s) - u(s)(t - s),$$

which is nonnegative because of the convexity of U. If we consider the Legendre transformation such as

$$U^*(t) = \sup_s \{ts - U(s)\}$$
$$= tu^{-1}(t) - U(u^{-1}(t)),$$

then the distance function is expressed as

$$d(s, t) = U^*(u(s)) + U(t) - u(s)t.$$

The distance $d(s, t) = 0$ if and only if $s = t$, which means that $D_U(\pi, \pi') = 0$ if and only if $\pi(x) = \pi'(x)$ (a.e. x).

U-divergence can be divided as follows:

$$D_U(\pi, \pi') = C_U(\pi, \pi') - H_U(\pi),$$

where

$$C_U(\pi, \pi') = -\sum_{x \in \mathcal{X}} \pi(x)\xi(\pi'(x)) + \sum_{x \in \mathcal{X}} U(\xi(\pi'(x)))$$
$$H_U(\pi) = C_U(\pi, \pi)$$
$$= -\sum_{x \in \mathcal{X}} \pi(x)\xi(\pi(x)) + \sum_{x \in \mathcal{X}} U(\xi(\pi(x))),$$

and $C_U(\pi, \pi')$ and $H_U(\pi)$ are the U-cross-entropy and U-entropy, respectively. U-divergence includes the Boltzmann–Gibbs–Shannon entropy when $U(t) = \exp(t)$:

$$H_U(\pi) = 1 - \sum_{x \in \mathcal{X}} \pi(x) \log(\pi(x))$$

This results in the Kullback–Leibler divergence as

$$D_U(\pi, \pi') = \sum_{x \in \mathcal{X}} \pi(x) \log \left(\frac{\pi(x)}{\pi'(x)} \right).$$

Similarly, if we consider

$$U_{(t)} = (1 + \beta t)^{(1+\beta)/\beta} / (1 + \beta)$$

we have

$$D_\beta(\pi, \pi') = -\frac{1}{\beta} \sum_{x \in \mathscr{X}} \pi(x)(\pi'(x)^\beta - \pi(x)^\beta) + \frac{1}{1+\beta} \sum_{x \in \mathscr{X}} \{\pi'(x)^{1+\beta} - \pi(x)^{1+\beta}\},$$

which is the β-divergence [1, 7]. It includes the Kullback–Leibler divergence, L_2 norm, and Itakura–Saito divergence because $\lim_{\beta \to 0} U_\beta(t) = \exp(t)$ and $D_1(\pi, \pi') = \sum_{x \in \mathscr{X}} (\pi(x) - \pi'(x))^2/2$ and $D_{-1} = \sum_{x \in \mathscr{X}} [\pi(x)/\pi'(x) - \log(\pi(x)/\pi'(x)) - 1]$. The last one is derived from the equation that

$$\log(t) = \lim_{a \to 0} \frac{t^a - 1}{a}.$$

Other divergences such as Csiszár f-divergence and $\alpha - \beta$ divergence are discussed in [2].

3.2 β-Maxent

The maximum β-entropy distribution [3] is given by

$$\pi_\beta(x|\lambda) = \frac{\left\{1 + \beta \lambda^\top f(x)\right\}^{\frac{1}{\beta}}}{Z_\lambda}, \tag{3.1}$$

where $Z_\lambda = \sum_{x \in \mathscr{X}} \{1 + \beta \lambda^\top f(x)\}^{1/\beta}$ and $f(x)$ is the feature vector or environmental variables. The coefficient λ is estimated by

$$\hat{\lambda}_\beta = \underset{\lambda \in \mathbb{R}^p}{\operatorname{argmin}} \, L_\beta(\pi_\beta(\cdot|\lambda)),$$

where

$$L_\beta(\pi(\cdot|\lambda)) = -\frac{1}{n} \sum_{i=1}^n \frac{\pi(x_i|\lambda)^\beta - 1}{\beta} + \frac{1}{1+\beta} \sum_{x \in \mathscr{X}} \pi(x|\lambda)^{1+\beta}. \tag{3.2}$$

This is the estimator by β-Maxent [5]. If the solution is unique, then $\hat{\lambda}_\beta$ satisfies the constraint

$$\mathbb{E}_{\pi_\beta(\cdot, \hat{\lambda}_\beta)}\{f(x)\} = \hat{f}.$$

$\mathbb{E}_{\pi_\beta}$ is the population mean over π_β and $\hat{f}$ is the sample mean of $f(x)$. In some cases, we can consider L_1-regularized β-loss to avoid the overfitting to the data

$$L_\beta^\alpha(\lambda) = L_\beta(\lambda) + \sum_{j=1}^{p} \alpha_j |\lambda_j|, \tag{3.3}$$

where $\alpha^\top = (\alpha_1, \ldots, \alpha_p)$ with $\alpha_j \geq 0$ for all j and $\lambda^\top = (\lambda_1, \ldots, \lambda_p)$. The estimator λ is given as

$$\hat{\lambda}_\beta^\alpha = \underset{\lambda \in \mathbb{R}^p}{\mathrm{argmin}}\, L_\beta^\alpha(\lambda).$$

3.2.1 Information Criterion for β-Divergence

If we consider a loss function rather than the log-likelihood for a data set D and a random variable z such as

$$L_D^b(\lambda) = -\sum_{i=1}^{n} \frac{\pi_\beta(x_i|\lambda)^b - 1}{b} + \frac{n}{1+b} \sum_{x \in \mathcal{X}} \pi_\beta(x|\lambda)^{1+b}$$

$$L_z^b(\lambda) = -\frac{\pi_\beta(z|\lambda)^b - 1}{b} + \frac{1}{1+b} \sum_{x \in \mathcal{X}} \pi_\beta(x|\lambda)^{1+b},$$

then the bias term becomes

$$\mathrm{bias}(G) = E_{G(D)}\Big[L_D^b(\hat{\lambda}_\beta) - n E_{G(z)}\{ L_z^b(\hat{\lambda}_\beta) \} \Big],$$

where $G(D)$ and $G(z)$ are probability distribution of D and z, respectively. After the derivation of the empirical version of $\mathrm{bias}(G)$ (Appendix), we have an information criterion such as

$$\mathrm{IC}_\beta^b = 2\{ L_D^b(\hat{\lambda}_\beta) - \mathrm{bias}(\hat{G}) \},$$

which reduces to GIC (generalized information criterion) [6] when b goes to 0.

3.2.2 Sequential-Update Algorithm for Estimation of $\hat{\lambda}_\beta$

---

1. Set $\lambda^{(1)^\top} = (0, \ldots, 0)$.
2. For $t = 1, \ldots, T$

   a. Choose $j^* \in \{1, \ldots, p\}$ and $\delta^* \in [-1, 1]$ such that

$$(j^*, \delta^*) = \underset{j, \delta}{\mathrm{argmin}}\, L_\beta\big(\lambda(j, \delta)\big), \tag{3.4}$$

where the jth component of $\lambda(j, \delta)$ are $\lambda_j^{(t)} + \delta$; the others are $\lambda_k^{(t)}$ ($k \neq j$).

b. Update the jth component of $\lambda^{(t)}$ as

$$\lambda_j^{(t+1)} = \begin{cases} \lambda_j^{(t)} + \delta^* & \text{if } j = j^* \\ \lambda_j^{(t)} & \text{otherwise} \end{cases} \tag{3.5}$$

3. Output $\hat{\lambda}_\beta = \lambda^{(T+1)}$.

The iteration step T is determined by GIC or IC_β^b.

3.3 *Bradypus Variegatus* Data Analysis

We compared the performance of Maxent and β-Maxent using *Bradypus variegatus* data, which is originally presented by [9]. It is available in the dismo package [4], which includes eight environmental variables from the WorldClim database (http://www.worldclim.org/bioclim): Annual Mean Temperature, Annual Precipitation, Precipitation of Wettest Quarter, Precipitation of Driest Quarter, Max Temperature of Warmest Month, Min Temperature of Coldest Month, Temperature Annual Range, and Mean Temperature of Wettest Quarter.

The tuning parameter of Maxent is the iteration number T; the optimal value of T determined by GIC is 96. For β-Maxent, there are two tuning parameters T and β, which are determined by GIC as well as IC_β^b, as shown in Fig. 3.1. Here, we fix the value of b to 0.5 as an anchor parameter as seen in [7]. Figure 3.1 shows the values of GIC in the left panel and those of IC_β^b in the right panel. Both criteria yield an optimal β of $\beta = 0.45$, and the iteration number are 17 and 15, respectively. This means that β-Maxent yields better model fitting than Maxent. The optimal values of β and T are similar for GIC or IC_β^b. However, there is a suboptimal value of GIC around $\beta = 0$, which is not quite different from the optimal value when $\beta = 0.45$. On the other hand, if we use IC_β^b, we can clearly identify the optimal value from Fig. 3.1. Hence, IC_β^b is preferable in practice.

The resultant estimated habitat maps of *Bradypus variegatus* generated by Maxent and β-Maxent are illustrated in Fig. 3.2. The presence locations are properly estimated with high probabilities for both methods, but there are differences in the values of estimated parameters $\hat{\lambda}$. For Maxent, we have $\hat{\lambda} = (0.000, 11.042, -4.189, -5.654, -1.004, 1.000, -11.998, 0.000)^\top$, whereas for β-Maxent, we have $\hat{\lambda} = (0.314, 0.747, 1.000, -0.816, 0.000, -0.692, -5.862, -0.378)^\top$. Hence, Annual Mean Temperature and Mean Temperature of Wettest Quarter are not included in Maxent; whereas, Max Temperature of Warmest Month is not in β-Maxent. The signs of the estimated coefficients are different for Precipitation of Wettest Quarter and Min Temperature of Coldest Month. The validity of the model should be further investigated, not only from a statistical viewpoint but also from an ecological one.

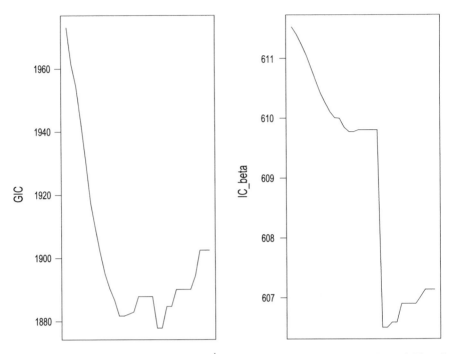

Fig. 3.1 Plots of GIC in the left panel and IC_β^b in the right panel against several values of β based on β-Maxent, where b is fixed to 0.5

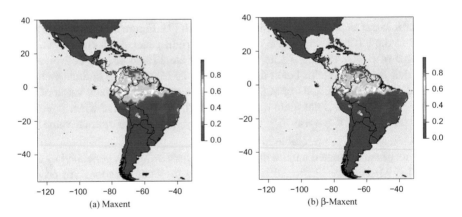

Fig. 3.2 Estimated habitat map of *Bradypus variegatus* data by Maxent (a) and β-Maxent, where presence locations are dotted by white circles

References

1. Basu A, Harris IR, Hjort N, Jones M (1998) Robust and efficient estimation by minimising a density power divergence. Biometrika 85:549–559
2. Cichocki A, Cruces S, Amari S (2011) Generalized alpha-beta divergences and their application to robust nonnegative matrix factorization. Entropy 13:134–170
3. Eguchi S, Komori O, Ohara A (2014) Duality of maximum entropy and minimum divergence. Entropy 16:3552–3572
4. Hijmans R, Phillips S, Leathwick J, Elith J (2013) Dismo: Species distribution modeling. R package version 9–3. http://CRAN.R-project.org/package=dismo
5. Komori O, Eguchi S (2014) Maximum power entropy method for ecological data analysis. In: Mohammad-Djafari A, Barbaresco F (eds) Bayesian inference and maximum entropy methods in science and engineering (Maxent2014). AIP publishing, New York, pp 337–344
6. Konishi S, Kitagawa G (1996) Generalised information criteria in model selection. Biometrika 83:875–890
7. Minami M, Eguchi S (2002) Robust blind source separation by beta divergence. Neural Comput 14:1859–1886
8. Murata N, Takenouchi T, Kanamori T, Eguchi S (2004) Information geometry of $\mathcal{U}$-boost and Bregman divergence. Neural Comput 16:1437–1481
9. Phillips SJ, Anderson RP, Schapire RE (2006) Maximum entropy modeling of species geographic distributions. Ecol Model 190:231–259

Chapter 4
Generalized T-Statistic

Abstract We discuss a statistical method for the classification problem with two groups $y = 0$ and $y = 1$. We envisage a situation in which the conditional distribution of $y = 0$ is well specified by a normal distribution, but the conditional distribution of $y = 1$ (rare observations in imbalanced data sets) is not well modeled by any specific distribution. Typically in a case-control study, the distribution in the control group can be assumed to be normal via an appropriate data transformation, whereas the distribution in the case group may depart from normality. In this situation, the maximum t-statistic for linear discrimination, or equivalently the Fisher's linear discriminant function, may not be optimal. We propose a class of generalized t-statistics and study asymptotic consistency and normality. The optimal generalized t-statistic in the sense of asymptotic variance is derived in a semi-parametric manner, and its statistical performance is confirmed in several numerical experiments.

Keywords Area under the ROC curve · Fisher's linear discriminant analysis · Kullback–Leibler divergence · T-statistics

4.1 Generalized T-Statistic

This chapter discusses a statistical method for a classification problem for two groups. For a binary class label $y \in \{0, 1\}$ and a covariate vector $x \in \mathbb{R}^p$, we envisage a statistical situation in which the conditional distribution of x given $y = 0$ is well specified by a normal distribution, but is not well modeled by a specific distribution when given $y = 1$.

In practice, we preliminarily perform a transformation for the data set of two groups such that only the data of $y = 0$ follow the normal distribution, leaving the distribution of $y = 1$ uncontrolled. If we could do a transformation that satisfied normality for both groups, then we could instead perform a simple classification task like Fisher's linear discriminant analysis. However, it is difficult to find such an idealistic transformation in the context of classification. Therefore, we discuss a situation where there exists an essential asymmetry for the distributions of the two groups.

© The Author(s), under exclusive licence to Springer Japan KK 2019
O. Komori and S. Eguchi, *Statistical Methods for Imbalanced Data in Ecological and Biological Studies*, JSS Research Series in Statistics,
https://doi.org/10.1007/978-4-431-55570-4_4

Let $\{x_{0i} : i = 1, \ldots, n_0\}$ be a sample of $y = 0$ and $\{x_{1j} : j = 1, \ldots, n_1\}$ be a sample of $y = 1$. Then, we propose a generalized t-statistic defined by

$$L_U(\beta) = \frac{1}{n_1} \sum_{j=1}^{n_1} U\left(\frac{\beta^{\mathrm{T}}(x_{1j} - \bar{x}_0)}{(\beta^{\mathrm{T}} S_0 \beta)^{1/2}}\right),$$

where U is a generator function, and $\bar{x}_y$ and S_y in general are the sample mean and the sample variance given y, respectively. The expectation of $L_U(\beta)$ is defined by

$$\mathbb{L}_U(\beta) = E_1\left\{U\left(\frac{\beta^{\mathrm{T}}(x - \mu_0)}{(\beta^{\mathrm{T}} \Sigma_0 \beta)^{1/2}}\right)\right\}, \tag{4.1}$$

where E_y, μ_y, and Σ_y denotes the conditional expectation, mean, and variance, respectively, given y. As mentioned above, we assume normality for the conditional distribution given $y = 0$ for the generalized t-statistic, e.g., $x_0 \sim N(\mu_0, \Sigma_0)$. This implies that the information of $y = 0$ population is simply reduced to the sufficient statistics $\bar{x}_0$ and S_0, whereas such sufficient statistics do not exist in $y = 1$ population.

Actually, in the analysis of cancer data based on gene expression data, a small part of observations of the disease group ($y = 1$) are clearly over- or down-expressed beyond the normality assumption. To treat such heterogeneity, several kinds of t-statistics have been proposed to individually detect genes that are useful in cancer studies [7, 10, 11]. Here, we consider such a problem in the classification framework in order to obtain an efficient discriminant function by combining multiple genes, rather than the two-sample test framework for single gene.

The main concern of this section is to characterize the generator function U, in which the conditional distribution of x given $y = 1$ is arbitrary. If we adopt an identity function $U(w) = w$, then the generalized t-statistic becomes the simple t-statistic standardized by S_0,

$$L_1(\beta) = \frac{\beta^{\mathrm{T}}(\bar{x}_1 - \bar{x}_0)}{(\beta^{\mathrm{T}} S_0 \beta)^{1/2}}. \tag{4.2}$$

When we take a cumulative function of a standard normal distribution $\Phi(w)$ as $U(w)$, the generalized t-statistic is viewed as the c-statistic (area under the ROC curve) due to the normality assumption for the $y = 0$ population,

$$L_\Phi(\beta) = \frac{1}{n_1} \sum_{j=1}^{n_1} \Phi\left(\frac{\beta^{\mathrm{T}}(x_{1j} - \bar{x}_0)}{(\beta^{\mathrm{T}} S_0 \beta)^{1/2}}\right), \tag{4.3}$$

which converges to $P(\beta^{\mathrm{T}} x_0 < \beta^{\mathrm{T}} x_1)$ as n_0 and n_1 go to infinity by a conditional expectation argument [9]. Hence, the generalized t-statistic is a natural extension of the common statistics such as the t-statistic and c-statistic. Moreover, the generalized t-statistic leads to the Fisher's linear discriminant function if we choose a specific quadratic function as U, which is investigated in the subsequent discussion.

Let us propose an estimator derived from the generalized t-statistic as follows:

$$\widehat{\beta}_U = \underset{\beta \in \mathbb{R}^p}{\text{argmax}} \ L_U(\beta).$$

We note that the maximizer of the generalized t-statistic in (4.1) has scale invariance in the sense that $L_U(\beta) = L_U(c\beta)$ for all $c > 0$. For this reason, we normalize $\widehat{\beta}_U$ to satisfy $\widehat{\beta}_U^{\mathrm{T}} S_0 \widehat{\beta}_U = 1$. In the most typical case of $U(w) = w$ as in (4.2), we have $\widehat{\beta}_U = S_0^{-1}(\bar{x}_1 - \bar{x}_0)/\{(\bar{x}_1 - \bar{x}_0)' S_0^{-1}(\bar{x}_1 - \bar{x}_0)\}^{1/2}$, which is almost surely convergent to

$$\beta_0 = \frac{\Sigma_0^{-1}(\mu_1 - \mu_0)}{\{(\mu_1 - \mu_0)^{\mathrm{T}} \Sigma_0^{-1}(\mu_1 - \mu_0)\}^{1/2}}. \tag{4.4}$$

4.2 Asymptotic Consistency

For simplicity of notation, we assume without loss of generality that $\mu_0 = (0, \ldots, 0)^{\mathrm{T}}$ and $\Sigma_0 = I$, where I is the $p \times p$ unit matrix. We also define two statistics $w = \beta_0^{\mathrm{T}} x$ and $g = Q_0 x$, where $Q_0 = I - \beta_0 \beta_0^{\mathrm{T}}$ for the investigation of the consistency of $\widehat{\beta}_U$ in the general case of U. In fact, we consider

(A) $E_1(g \mid w = a) = 0$ for all $a \in \mathbb{R}$.

(B) $\text{var}_1(g \mid w = a) = Q_0$ for all $a \in \mathbb{R}$,

where var_y denotes the conditional variance of x given y. As a typical case, a mislabel model is given as

$$p_1(x) = (1 - \varepsilon)\phi(x, v_1, I) + \varepsilon\phi(x, 0, I), \tag{4.5}$$

where p_y is a probability density function of x given y and $\phi(x, \mu, \Sigma)$ denotes a normal density function with mean μ and variance Σ. We note that $(1 - \varepsilon)v_1 = \mu_1$, where ε is the mislabel probability describing the model uncertainty for $P(x \mid y = 1)$. The larger the value of ε, the more uncertain labeling of $y = 0$ or $y = 1$ in the population.

We note that this mislabel model (4.5) satisfies (A) and (B) because w and g are stochastically independent under the normal distribution.

In addition to Assumptions (A) and (B), we need a condition under which the Hessian matrix of $\mathbb{L}_U(\beta)$, denoted by $H_U(\beta)$, at $\beta = \beta_0$ should be negative definite in order to show the consistency of $\hat{\beta}_U$, where $\mathbb{L}_U(\beta)$ and β_0 are defined as in (4.1) and (4.4), respectively. Actually, from Assumption (A) and (B), $H_U(\beta_0) = E_1\{U''(w) - U'(w)w\}Q_0$, so this assumption is equivalent to

(C) $E_1[U''(w) - U'(w)w] < 0.$

Note that under Assumptions (A), (B), and (C), $\widehat{\beta}_U$ is asymptotically consistent with β_0 for any U.

If we consider a semi-parametric model for any strictly increasing function $\psi(\cdot)$ such as

$$\psi\left\{\frac{p_1(x)}{p_0(x)}\right\} = c + \beta^\top x, \tag{4.6}$$

then we observe that the target parameter β_0 is proportional to β in (4.6) and both assumptions (A) and (B) hold [6]. In this case, the estimated linear function $\widehat{\beta}_U^\top x$ converges to $\beta_0^\top x$ which has one-to-one correspondence to $p_1(x)/p_0(x)$, and thus is Bayes risk consistent. This semi-parametric model is extended and further investigated by [1].

Hence, β_0 can be regarded as the target value of the estimator $\hat{\beta}_U$ for any generator function U such as those defined in (4.2) and (4.3), and introduced in the subsequent discussion.

4.3 Asymptotic Normality and Optimality

In the case that the conditional random covariate given $y = 0$ and $y = 1$ are both distributed normally with the common variance, the property of asymptotic variance of the coefficients of the Fisher's linear discriminant function was fully investigated by [5] in comparison with that of the logistic regression. The result is extended to non-normal distribution's case of some parametric model by [8]. Here, we consider the asymptotic variance of $\hat{\beta}_U$ with more general assumptions. It turns out that the asymptotic variance is expressed as a function of the first derivative of U denoted by U', and that the optimal-U function achieving the minimum asymptotic variance has a close relationship with a probability density function of w given $y = 1$ denoted by $f_1(w)$.

Under Assumptions (A) and (B), $n_1^{1/2}(\widehat{\beta}_U - \beta_0)$ is asymptotically distributed as $N(0, \Sigma_U)$, where

$$\Sigma_U = c_U(Q_0)^-,$$

$$c_U = \frac{E_1\{U'(w)^2\} + \pi_1/\pi_0\left[E_1\{U'(w)w\}\right]^2 + \pi_1/\pi_0\left[E_1\{U'(w)\}\right]^2}{\left[E_1\{U''(w)\} - E_1\{U'(w)w\}\right]^2},$$

where $\pi_0 = P(y = 0)$, $\pi_1 = P(y = 1)$ and $(Q_0)^-$ is the generalized inverse of Q_0 [6].

The asymptotic variance consists of a scalar c_U and a matrix Q_0, which is independent of U. Hence, the minimization of Σ_U is reduced to the functional minimization of c_U with respect to U'. The optimal-U function under Assumptions (A) and (B) has the following form:

$$U_{\text{opt}}(w) = \log \frac{f_1(w)}{\phi(w, m, s^2)},$$

where $m = E(w)$ and $s^2 = \text{var}(w)$ [6].

Remark 4.1 The expectation of the generalized t-statistic based on U_{opt} is equivalent to the Kullback–Leibler divergence and is given as

$$\mathbb{L}_{U_{\text{opt}}}(\beta) = \int f_1(w) \log \frac{f_1(w)}{\phi(w, m, s^2)} dw.$$

That is, the maximization of the generalized t-statistic is considered as the maximization of the Kullback–Leibler divergence.

Remark 4.2 When μ_0 and Σ_0 are known, the optimal-U function is reduced to the logarithm of the likelihood ration of the probability density function of w given $y = 1$ and $y = 0$, respectively. That is, $U_{\text{opt}}(w) = \log\{f_1(w)/\phi(w, 0, 1)\}$.

Remark 4.3 When x_1 is normally distributed, we have $f_1(w) = \phi(w, m_1, s_1^2)$, where $m_1 = E_1(w)$, $s_1^2 = \text{var}_1(w)$. Then, the optimal U has the following form up to constant factors:

$$U(w) = -(w - c)^2, \tag{4.7}$$

where $c = \{\pi_0 + \pi_1(s_1^2 + m_1^2)\}/(\pi_1 m_1)$.

The maximization of $L_U(\beta)$ based on U defined in (4.7) is not straightforward because c_0 contains m_1 and s_1^2, which depend on unknown parameter β_0. Hence, we apply a fixed-point iteration for $t = 1, \ldots, T$:

$$\beta_t = \underset{\beta}{\text{argmax}} \, L_{\hat{U}_{\beta_{t-1}}}(\beta),$$

where $\hat{U}_{\beta_{t-1}}(w) = -(w - \hat{c}_{\beta_{t-1}})^2$, $\hat{c}_{\beta_{t-1}} = [\hat{\pi}_0 + \hat{\pi}_1\{\hat{s}_{1,t-1}^2 + \hat{m}_{1,t-1}^2\}]/\{\hat{\pi}_1 \hat{m}_{1,t-1}\}$, $\hat{\pi}_0 = n_0/n$, $\hat{\pi}_1 = n_1/n$, $\hat{m}_{1,t-1} = \beta_{t-1}^T(\bar{x}_1 - \bar{x}_0)/(\beta_{t-1}^T S_0 \beta_{t-1})$, and $s_{1,t-1}^2 = \beta_{t-1}^T S_1 \beta_{t-1}/(\beta_{t-1}^T S_0 \beta_{t-1})$. This procedure will be extended and investigated in detail for the general case in the next subsection. Here, we show the close relationship between the quadratic U function in (4.7) and the Fisher's linear discriminant function.

Proposition 4.1 *If $\beta_\infty = \underset{\beta}{\text{argmax}} \, L_{\hat{U}_{\beta_\infty}}(\beta)$, then it holds that*

$$\beta_\infty \propto (\hat{\pi}_0 S_0 + \hat{\pi}_1 S_1)^{-1}(\bar{x}_1 - \bar{x}_0).$$

That is, the estimator based on the quadratic function in (4.7) is proportional to the
slope vector of the Fisher's linear discriminant function.

The generalized t-statistic is defined by the standardization based only on the
sample variance S_0, whereas the slope vector of the Fisher's linear discriminant
function involves the term depending on S_1 as given in Proposition 4.1. We note that
the quadratic term in $U(w)$ defined in (4.7) has connection to the dependence on S_1,
because

$$\sum_{j=1}^{n_1} w_{1j}^2 = \frac{\beta_t^T\{S_1 + (\bar{x}_1 - \bar{x}_0)(\bar{x}_1 - \bar{x}_0)^T\}\beta_t}{\beta_t^T S_0 \beta_t},$$

where $w_{1j} = \beta_t^T(x_{1j} - \bar{x}_0)/(\beta_t^T S_0 \beta_t)^{1/2}$.

Note that the slope of the Fisher's linear discriminant function can be calculated
without any computation of the inverse matrix of $\hat{\pi}_0 S_0 + \hat{\pi}_1 S_1$ in the algorithm.

4.4 Algorithm for $\widehat{\beta}_{U_{\text{Opt}}}$

The optimal U consists of the probability density function w given $y = 1$ and its mean
and variance. Hence, in order to derive $\widehat{\beta}_{U_{\text{opt}}}$, we have to maximize the generalized
t-statistic $L_U(\beta)$ as well as estimate U_{opt} at the same time in the following algorithm:

---

1. Set $\beta_1 = S_0^{-1}(\bar{x}_1 - \bar{x}_0)$.
2. For $t = 2, \ldots, T$

    a. Estimate $\hat{U}(w)$ based on β_{t-1}.
    b. Update β_{t-1} to β_t as

$$\beta_t = \underset{\beta \in \mathbb{R}^p}{\text{argmax}} \frac{1}{n_1} \sum_{j=1}^{n_1} \hat{U}\left\{\frac{\beta^T(x_{1j} - \bar{x}_0)}{(\beta^T S_0 \beta)^{1/2}}\right\}.$$

3. Output $\widehat{\beta}_U = \beta_T/(\beta_T^T S_0 \beta_T)^{1/2}$

For estimation of $\hat{U}(w) = \log\{\hat{f}_1(w)/\phi(w, \hat{m}, \hat{s}^2)\}$ in Step 2.a, we calculate $\hat{m} = \hat{\pi}_1\hat{m}_1$ and $\hat{s}^2 = \hat{\pi}_0 + \hat{\pi}_1\hat{s}_1^2 + \hat{\pi}_0\hat{\pi}_1\hat{m}_1^2$, where $\hat{m}_1 = \beta_{t-1}^T(\bar{x}_1 - \bar{x}_0)/(\beta_{t-1}^T S_0 \beta_{t-1})^{1/2}$
and $\hat{s}_1^2 = \beta_{t-1}^T S_1 \beta_{t-1}/\beta_{t-1}^T S_0 \beta_{t-1}$, respectively.

Then, we estimate $\hat{f}_1(w)$ using $w_{1j} = \beta_{t-1}^T(x_{1j} - \bar{x}_0)/(\beta_{t-1}^T S_0 \beta_{t-1})^{1/2}$ $(j = 1, \ldots, n_1)$, based on the kernel density estimation [3, 4]. That is,

$$\hat{f}_1(w) = \frac{1}{n_1} \sum_{j=1}^{n_1} \phi(w, w_{1j}, \hat{h}),$$

where $\hat{h}$ is the estimated bandwidth. The form of $\hat{f}_1(w)$ determines that of the optimal $\hat{U}(w)$. If it is estimated to be one-component normal density, $\hat{U}(w)$ would be the quadratic function defined in (4.7). Also, it gets close to a linear function if π_0 is very small such that $\hat{s}^2$ is approximately equal to $\hat{\sigma}_{1,w}$.

In this way, the heterogeneity of the population of $y = 1$ is flexibly captured by $\hat{f}_1(w)$, although the homogeneity assumed in a population of $y = 0$ is simply summarized by $\bar{x}_0$ and S_0. The stopping time T is defined to satisfy that $\|\beta_T - \beta_{T-1}\|/\|\beta_{T-1}\| < 10^{-5}$ or to be 30 if β_T does not converge, where $\|\cdot\|$ denotes the Euclid norm.

4.5 U-Lasso

We define the U-lasso by adding an L_1-regularization term such as

$$L_U^\lambda(\beta) = L_U(\beta) - \lambda \sum_{k=1}^{p} |\beta_k|, \qquad (4.8)$$

where $\beta = (\beta_1, \ldots, \beta_p)^\top$, and λ is a nonnegative parameter that controls the shrinkage of β. This is implemented by the ULasso package by [6].

```
> install.packages("ULasso_1.0.tar.gz",type="source",repo=NULL)
> library(ULasso)
> help(ULasso)
```

We then load the asthmatic data [2] of group X.

```
> data(dat.x)
```

Then, we estimate β based on the linear-U, auc-U, quadratic-U and optimal-U functions.

```
> x=dat.x
> label=x$lab
> x$lab=NULL
> y=label=="asthmatic"
# estimation of beta based on the linear-U function
> ulasso(x,y,type="linear")
# estimation of beta based on the auc-U function
> ulasso(x,y,type="auc")
# estimation of beta based on the quadratic-U function
> ulasso(x,y,type="quad")
# used for estimation of optimal-U function
```

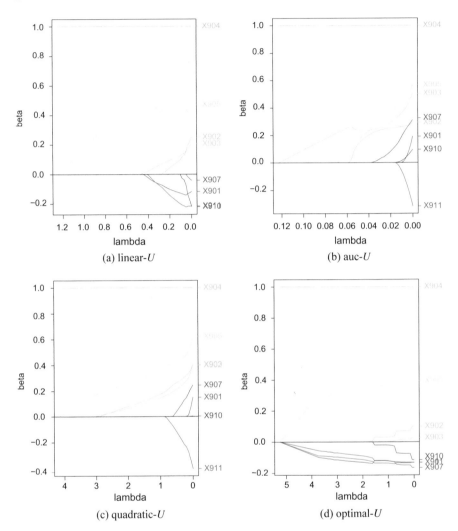

Fig. 4.1 Solution paths by linear-U, auc-U, quadratic-U, and optimal-U lasso

```
> library(ks)
# estimation of beta based on the optimal-U function
> ulasso(x,y)
```

The resultant path plots are illustrated in Fig. 4.1. The coefficient of the anchor
variable X904, which is the most informative in determining the class label, is fixed
to be 1. The next important variable turns out to be X905 based on linear-, quadratic-
and optimal-U, where X901, X907, and X911 are also estimated to be important for
optimal-U. For further analysis of the asthmatic data, see [6].

References

1. Baek S, Komori O, Ma Y (2018) An optimal semiparametric method for two-group classification. Scand J Stat 45:806–846
2. Dottorini T, Sole G, Nunziangeli L, Baldracchini F, Senin N, Mazzoleni G, Proietti C, Balaci L, Crisanti A (2011) Serum IgE reactivity profiling in an asthma affected cohort. PLoS ONE 6:e22319
3. Duong T, Hazelton ML (2003) Plug-in bandwidth matrices for bivariate kernel density estimation. Nonparametric Stat 15:17–30
4. Duong T (2007) ks: Kernel density estimation and kernel discriminant analysis for multivariate data in R. J Stat Softw 21:1–16
5. Efron B (1975) The efficiency of logistic regression compared to normal discriminant analysis. J Am Stat Assoc 70:892–898
6. Komori O, Eguchi S, Copas JB (2015) Generalized t-statistic for two-group classification. Biometrics 71:404–416
7. Lian H (2008) MOST: detecting cancer differential gene expression. Biostatistics 9:411–418
8. O'Neill TJ (1980) The general distribution of the error rate of a classification procedure with application to logistic regression discrimination. J Am Stat Assoc 75:154–160
9. Su JQ, Liu JS (1993) Linear combinations of multiple diagnostic markers. J Am Stat Assoc 88:1350–1355
10. Tibshirani R, Hastie T (2007) Outlier sums for differential gene expression analysis. Biostatistics 8:2–8
11. Wu B (2007) Cancer outlier differential gene expression detection. Biostatistics 8:566–575

Chapter 5
Machine Learning Methods for Imbalanced Data

Abstract We discuss high-dimensional data analysis in the framework of pattern recognition and machine learning, including single-component analysis and clustering analysis. Several boosting methods for tackling imbalances in sample sizes are investigated.

Keywords Adaboost · SMOTEBoost · pAUCBoost · Machine learning

5.1 High-Dimensional Data Analysis

5.1.1 Single-Component Analysis

The first step of high-dimensional data analysis with $p \gg n$, such as gene expression data, is ranking of p individual variables based on how closely they relate to the phenotype or class label, e.g., disease or non-disease. This can be referred to as single-component analysis, and is performed as a preprocessing step to extract some useful variables, for which statistical methods such as boosting are employed [4, 6, 15, 32]. When the phenotype is binary, the single-component analysis is reduced to the two-sample test. Typical examples are Student's t-statistic (S_t), Welch's statistic (W_t), and C-statistic (C).

Let $\{\boldsymbol{x}_{-i} \in \mathbb{R}^p : i = 1, \ldots, n_-\}$ and $\{\boldsymbol{x}_{+j} \in \mathbb{R}^p : j = 1, \ldots, n_+\}$ be samples for class label $y = -1$ and $y = +1$, respectively. Then the statistic S_t for the kth element of $x^{(k)}$ ($k = 1, \ldots, p$) consisting of $x_{-i}^{(k)}$ and $x_{+j}^{(k)}$, is expressed as

$$S_t(x^{(k)}) = (\bar{x}_+^{(k)} - \bar{x}_-^{(k)}) \bigg/ \sqrt{\frac{n_- + n_+}{n_- n_+ (n_- + n_+ - 2)} \Big[(n_- - 1)\{s_-^{(k)}\}^2 + (n_+ - 1)\{s_+^{(k)}\}^2 \Big]},$$

where $\bar{x}_-^{(k)}$ and $\bar{x}_+^{(k)}$ are sample means; $s_-^{(k)}$ and $s_+^{(k)}$ are sample variances Note that this statistic assumes a normal distribution as well as equal variance in general. When sample sizes n_- and n_+ are large enough, the normality assumption approximately holds. However, it is often the case that the covariance of each class is not equal. In

O. Komori and S. Eguchi, *Statistical Methods for Imbalanced Data in Ecological and Biological Studies*, JSS Research Series in Statistics,
https://doi.org/10.1007/978-4-431-55570-4_5

that case Welch's statistic is alternatively used:

$$W_t(x^{(k)}) = (\bar{x}_+^{(k)} - \bar{x}_-^{(k)}) \Big/ \sqrt{\frac{\{s_-^{(k)}\}^2}{n_-} + \frac{\{s_+^{(k)}\}^2}{n_+}}.$$

When normality is not satisfied, the nonparametric statistic C is used,

$$C(x^{(k)}) = \frac{1}{n_- n_+} \sum_{i=1}^{n_-} \sum_{j=1}^{n_+} \mathrm{H}\left(x_{+j}^{(k)} - x_{-i}^{(k)}\right), \tag{5.1}$$

where $\mathrm{H}(z)$ is the Heaviside function: $\mathrm{H}(z) = 1$ if $z > 0$, $1/2$ if $z = 0$, and 0 otherwise. This is called the area under the receiver operating curve (AUC), which is equivalent to the Mann–Whitney or Wilcoxon statistic [16]. From the definitions above, we can see that S_t and S_t are invariant under an affine transformation such as $x \mapsto ax + b$ $(a > 0)$, and that C is also unchangeable to a monotonically increasing transformation. Therefore, in the ranking of variables standardized based on the means and standard deviations, we have the same results whatever statistics we use. However, for log transformations which are often used to preprocess gene expression data, the ranking of variables is unchanged only for C. Note that in this ranking, no regard is given to the interaction or mutual effects among variables. That is, the variables selected by the ranking method above do not necessarily guarantee the best combination for predicting the class label $y \in \{-1, +1\}$. As an approach to tackling this problem, boosting methods based on C were proposed by [21, 22].

5.1.2 Clustering

As discussed in the last subsection, the single-component analysis is an important step for grasping the association of the gene with the phenotype in statistical analyses with $p \gg n$. However, it cannot capture any function for multiple genes, including interactions over genes. We need to get a brief map for correlations among genes and phenotype, in which the clustering method works effectively to give basic information and understandings of the data. In particular, the heat map generated by the clustering gives an intuitive understanding of the correlations of genes [8]. For example, the subtype of breast cancer and treatment effect are closely related, and clustering yields a clear separation among subtypes [30].

There are several choices of distance functions in clustering algorithms to accommodate the object of the analysis in both hierarchical and partition paradigms, including the Euclidean metric and the Pearson correlation coefficient [5]. The Euclidean metric is appropriate for measuring expression levels among subjects, whereas the Pearson correlation coefficient is appropriate for measuring the mutual directions for expression vectors over the subjects. The Spearman rank correlation coefficient is an alternative to the Pearson correlation coefficient that is robust for outliers. For the hierarchical approach, there is the nearest neighbor method, the furthest neighbor method, the group average method, and Ward's method. For the partition approach, there are k-means, fuzzy c-means, and the model-based clustering. Recently, many novel methods for clustering have been proposed, including functional data clustering and kernel clustering in reproducing kernel Hilbert spaces; however, we note that there is no optimal procedure for the clustering in which optimality depends on the objective of the data analysis. We have to select one of the most appropriate procedures in accordance with the objective and goal of data analysis.

5.2 Framework for Pattern Recognition

Machine learning, which originated in the late twentieth century, is a relatively new field outside of the statistical community. The main paradigm is learning from data, which is almost equivalent to inference based on data in the statistical sense. Thus, several approaches are common to machine learning and statistics, and are shared with artificial intelligence, data mining, and so forth. In this era of information-intensive societies, there exist mature communities with global networks, in which large-scale datasets are created and shared in our daily lives. Furthermore, these data analyses and algorithms have become widespread because of the useful statistical software such as S and R, which help us share understandings of such data sets in various scientific fields. Such developments are made over several areas in a cross-sectional manner, rather than in a specifically oriented manner. In the field of statistical pattern recognition, there have been multiple developments via learning algorithms proposed in several directions of machine learning [9, 10, 18, 28, 29].

In the field of statistics, statistical pattern recognition has been established through Fisher's linear discriminant analysis and logistic discriminant analysis, in which new proposals were derived from machine learning paradigm and discussion on the statistical properties for the proposed methods [2, 12, 23]. Previously, areas of pattern recognition are specialized in applied areas such as image, speech, character recognition. In the last two decades, there has been a substantial change in approaches to pattern recognition, in which two powerful methods of support vector machine (SVM) and AdaBoost algorithm have enlarged the universal applicability for various problems. SVM flexibly learns nonlinearity of data structure without over-learning by employing a sound theory in reproducing kernel Hilbert space. SVM is defined by maximization of the margin employing mathematical programming in which the kernel trick is cleverly employed to achieve nonlinearity for the decision boundary. The kernel method is applicable to the situation in which almost conventional multivariate analysis is used as in a linear model. The AdaBoost algorithm enables effective learning by combining various learning machines according to an empirical training set, so that the combined machine has much greater predictive power. Here, "learning machine" denotes a unit with output from the feature vector to a class label, which is a classifier in statistics. A comparison of the performance of SVM and AdaBoost is not important because AdaBoost can integrate different SVMs into a powerful machine, and the exponential loss function deriving AdaBoost can be implemented as a kernel machine equivalent to the SVM. In this sense, these approaches are not competitive, but are instead compatible and strengthen each other's weak points, opening a new path to performing pattern recognition in a unified manner.

Statistical pattern recognition reflects the structure of our brain when making a prediction in an instinctive way. The framework is simple such that there are a feature vector x and a class label y. Here, we confine ourselves to a case in which y is binary with values $\{-1, +1\}$. The function h of x into y is called a classifier. When x and y are viewed as input and output, the classifier is also said to be a learning machine. The goal for pattern recognition is to construct an efficient learning machine, which is usually given by a discriminant function $F(x, y)$ as follows:

$$h(x) = \operatorname*{argmax}_{y \in \{-1, +1\}} F(x, y), \qquad (5.2)$$

where argmax denotes the maximizer. In the binary classification, we conventionally define $F(x) = F(x, +1) - F(x, -1)$, which implies the classifier in (5.2) can be written as

$$h(x) = \operatorname{sign} F(x),$$

where sign denotes a sign function. Let $D_{\text{train}} = \{(x_1, y_1), \cdots, (x_n, y_n)\}$ be a training data set. Then, the Fisher's linear discriminant function and the logistic discriminant function have both the linear form

$$F(x, \beta) = \beta_1^\top x + \beta_0 \qquad (5.3)$$

so that the vector $\beta = (\beta_1^\top, \beta_0)^\top$ is given by learning from D_{train}. Here, the Fisher's linear discriminant function is derived by the estimative distribution, whereas the logistic discriminant function is directly given by the maximum likelihood for the conditional model [7].

5.2.1 AdaBoost

In a common context in bioinformatics, our goal is to predict a treatment effect for cancer patients. For example, consider a setting in which p gene levels $x = (x^{(1)}, \ldots, x^{(p)})^\top$ are observed for n subjects. In this situation, AdaBoost usually employs a set of learning machines defined by the kth gene expression $x^{(k)}$, such that

$$h^{(k)}(x) = \begin{cases} +1 \text{ if } x^{(k)} > b^{(k)} \\ -1 \text{ if } x^{(k)} \le b^{(k)}, \end{cases} \qquad (5.4)$$

where $b^{(k)}$ denotes the threshold value. Thus, the machine $h^{(k)}$ is the simplest machine neglecting all other gene expression but the kth one, which is called a stump for the kth gene. If we consider all possible threshold values, the number of stumps becomes extremely large. One element of the set never has high performance, but the set has exhaustive information from the gene expression levels. Our goal is to look for an efficient combination from the set via AdaBoost. More precisely, we extract T stumps $h_1^*(x), \ldots, h_T^*(x)$ in the hull of the stump set $\mathcal{H}$, so that the discriminant function linearly combined is decided sequentially:

$$F_T(x) = \sum_{t=1}^{T} \alpha_t h_t^*(x).$$

In a practical algorithm, we define the exponential loss function

$$L_{\exp}(F) = \frac{1}{n} \sum_{i=1}^{n} \exp\{-y_i F(x_i)\}$$

such that the sequential minimization for the exponential loss function from $F_{t-1}(x)$ to $F_t(x) = F_{t-1}(x) + \alpha_t h_t^*(x)$ is given by

$$h_t^* = \operatorname*{argmin}_{h \in \mathcal{H}} \nabla L_{\exp}(F_{t-1}, h) \tag{5.5}$$

$$\alpha_t = \operatorname*{argmin}_{\alpha \in (0, \infty)} L_{\exp}(F_{t-1} + \alpha h_t^*), \tag{5.6}$$

where $F_0(x) = 0$ and

$$\nabla L_{\exp}(F, h) = \frac{\partial}{\partial \alpha} L_{\exp}(F + \alpha h) \Big|_{\alpha=0},$$

which is not the same as the original definition but they are equivalent.

In accordance with this, AdaBoost is a gradient algorithm for minimization of the exponential loss function with respect to (h, α), in which the functional part h is different from the usual one. The most characteristic step is (5.5), in which the optimal solution shows good performance if the learning set $\mathcal{H}$ is sufficiently rich [23]. In any step, the best stump h_{t+1}^* is selected to have a minimum weighted error rate over all the stumps, which is totally different from the last candidate h_t^*. Thus, a drastic change in the weight reveals a discovery of a new characteristic by updating weights.

Within the machine learning community, there has been a historical controversy on a basic question of whether we can build a powerful machine combining weak machines (see [28]). In fact, among several promising proposals, the AdaBoost shows a universal learnability for problems in pattern recognition [9, 10, 29].

Usually, we set $F_0(x) = 0$ as the initial condition and build a stopping rule, e.g., monitoring the cross-validated loss function, so that we terminate the algorithm at

$t = T$, cf. Zhang2005. In this way, the final form of discriminant function is given by

$$F(x) = \sum_{t=1}^{T} \alpha_t h_t^*(x), \qquad (5.7)$$

which is the same as the classical discriminant function (5.3) in the sense of linearity, but the set of stumps in (5.7) are selected according to the learning process. In summary, a class label y with a feature vector x is predicted by majority vote for voters $h_t^*(x)$ with the weights α_t $(t = 1, \ldots, T)$.

In principle, the boosting method does not directly learn from the feature vector, instead of combining the best machine with the integrated machine in the current step. Consequently, the method does not suffer from the problem of '$p \gg n$' [13]. For an extreme case of $p \gg n$ the group boosting method is proposed in [31].

5.2.2 SMOTEBoost

SMOTEBoost is a boosting method that combines AdaBoost [9] and SMOTE, in which observations of minority class are oversampled. AdaBoost iteratively reweights observations in such a way that it focuses on observations that are hard to correctly classify in the previous iteration step. The algorithm is as follows [17]:

---

1. Set the weights as $w_1(i) = \frac{1}{n}$ for $i = 1, \ldots, n$.
2. For $t = 1, \ldots, T$,

    a. Prepare a set of stumps $\mathscr{H}_t$ based on the oversampled data $x_1, \ldots, x_n$, $x_{n+1}, \ldots, x_{n'}$ $(n' > n)$
    b. Compute the weighted error

    $$\varepsilon_t(h) = \frac{\sum_{i=1}^{n} w_t(i) I(y_i \neq h(x_i))}{\sum_{i=1}^{n} w_t(i)}$$

    c. Select a weak learner among $\mathscr{H}_t$

    $$h_t = \underset{h \in \mathscr{H}_t}{\operatorname{argmin}} \ \varepsilon_t(h)$$

    d. Calculate the coefficient

    $$\alpha_t = \frac{1}{2} \log \frac{1 - \varepsilon_t(h_t)}{\varepsilon_t(h_t)}$$

e. Update the weight

$$w_{t+1}(i) = w_t(i) \exp(-\alpha_t h_t(x_i) y_i).$$

3. Output $F(x) = \sum_{t=1}^{T} \alpha_t h_t(x)$.

We classify observations using $\text{sign}(F(x))$, where positive and negative values indicate the minority ($y = 1$) and majority ($y = -1$) classes, respectively. Regression trees and natural cubic splines are also used instead of stumps [11, 22]. In the AdaBoost algorithm, the set of stumps $\mathscr{H}$ is uniquely determined based on the original data $x_1, \ldots, x_n$, so this step (a) can be usually moved to the outside of the iteration process $t = 1, \ldots, T$. However, in the SMOTEBoost algorithm, $\mathscr{H}_t$ is constructed by the oversampled data $x_1, \ldots, x_n, x_{n+1}, \ldots, x_{n'}$ ($n' > n$), which depends on the iteration step t. This newly introduced step reduces the bias due to the class imbalance [3]. Other boosting methods for imbalanced data have been well summarized in [14].

5.2.3 RareBoost

RareBoost [19] is a boosting method that modifies the AdaBoost algorithm. In AdaBoost, the weighted error is calculated to produce the coefficient α_t, so it is affected by imbalance of the class labels. In RareBoost, the coefficients are separately calculated according to the sign of the stump $h_t(x_i)$. In fact, the coefficients of α_t^p and α_t^n are calculated as

$$\alpha_t^p = \frac{1}{2} \log \frac{TP_t}{FP_t}$$

$$\alpha_t^n = \frac{1}{2} \log \frac{TN_t}{FN_t},$$

where

$$TP_t = \sum_{i:h_t(x_i)=1, y_i=1} w_t(i)h_t(x_i), \quad FP_t = \sum_{i:h_t(x_i)=1, y_i=-1} w_t(i)h_t(x_i)$$

$$TN_t = \sum_{i:h_t(x_i)=-1, y_i=-1} w_t(i)h_t(x_i), \quad FN_t = \sum_{i:h_t(x_i)=-1, y_i=1} w_t(i)h_t(x_i).$$

The weights are also separately updated for i such that $h_t(x_i) = 1$ and i such that $h_t(x_i) = -1$ as

$$w_{t+1}(i) = w_t(i) \exp(-\alpha_t^p h_t(x_i) y_i),$$
$$w_{t+1}(i) = w_t(i) \exp(-\alpha_t^n h_t(x_i) y_i),$$

respectively. The final output is

$$F(x) = \sum_{t:h_t(x)=1} \alpha_t^p h_t(x) + \sum_{t:h_t(x)=-1} \alpha_t^n h_t(x).$$

5.2.4 AUCBoost

A boosting method that is designed for maximization of AUC [21] assumes the following model:

$$F(x) = F_1(x^{(1)}) + \cdots + F_p(x^{(p)}),$$

where $x = (x^{(1)}, \ldots, x^{(p)})'$. In general, the plot of $F(x^{(k)})$ against $x^{(k)}$ is called score plot [20] or coordinate function [12]. This model allows for nonlinearity of $F(x)$ to improve the classification accuracy as well as puts importance on the interpretability of the effects of each x^k, which is essential for understanding the relationship with class label y (e.g., disease vs. non-disease).

Since the AUC has a probabilistic interpretation as in [1], it can be expressed using probability densities for $y = -1$ and $y = +1$ as

$$\text{AUC}(F) = \int \int H(F(x_+) - F(x_-))g_-(x_-)g_+(x_+)dx_-dx_+,$$

where $H(\cdot)$ is the Heaviside function. Similarly, the empirical AUC using $\{x_{-i} : i = 1, \ldots, n_-\}$ and $\{x_{+j} : j = 1, \ldots, n_+\}$ is given by

$$\overline{\text{AUC}}(F) = \frac{1}{n_- n_+} \sum_{i=1}^{n_-} \sum_{j=1}^{n_+} H(F(x_{+j}) - F(x_{-i})). \tag{5.8}$$

If we consider $F(x^{(k)})$ in (5.8), it reduces to the C statistic defined in (5.1). Therefore, the empirical AUC above is regarded as a generalization of the C statistic. However, in the optimization procedure, we face difficulties because the empirical AUC is a sum of the noncontinuous function $H(\cdot)$. That is, we cannot apply the gradient method which is widely used due to its efficiency. The optimization method was first proposed by [26, 27], which used a grid search to find the optimal function $F(x)$, assuming that $F(x)$ is a linear function with a few variables ($p = 2$). To avoid difficulties with the optimization, [24, 33] proposed a surrogate function that smooths the empirical AUC so that it can be differentiable. The surrogate functions for the AUC and empirical AUC based on the standard normal distribution function $\Phi(\cdot)$ are given as

$$\mathrm{AUC}_\sigma(F) = \int\int \mathrm{H}_\sigma(F(x_+) - F(x_-))g_-(x_-)g_+(x_+)dx_-dx_+.$$

$$\overline{\mathrm{AUC}}_\sigma(F) = \frac{1}{n_-n_+}\sum_{i=1}^{n_-}\sum_{j=1}^{n_+}\mathrm{H}_\sigma(F(x_{+j}) - F(x_{-i})),$$

where $\mathrm{H}_\sigma(z) = \Phi(z/\sigma)$. A smaller value of σ means A better approximation of the AUC. Also, the relationship between the AUC and empirical AUC is given by

$$\sup_F \mathrm{AUC}_\sigma(F) = \mathrm{AUC}(\Lambda),$$

where $\Lambda(x) = g_+(x)/g_-(x)$. This provides a justification for the use of the empirical AUC rather than the AUC. Note that this equation holds even if we use a sigmoid function as in [24, 33], instead of $\mathrm{H}_\sigma(\cdot)$.

5.2.5   pAUC Boosting

As seen in the definition of the AUC, the overall range of FPR and TPR is taken into consideration. However, in the analysis of medical data, we often focus on a limited range of FPR or TPR because of its medical or biological background. For example, in disease screening, the targeted population consists of mainly healthy subjects, and we have many more controls ($y = -1$) than cases ($y = +1$). In this context, a large FPR value results in a large number of controls undergoing unnecessary treatment. By contrast, if we are diagnosing subjects with severe disease, it is preferable to keep TPR as high as possible. To deal with these situations, the partial area under the ROC (pAUC) curve has recently attracted attention. The authors of [27] proposed a method for maximization of the pAUC based on two variables. To accommodate a large number of variables, the authors of [33] considered a surrogate function for pAUC in a similar way to the case of the AUC, in order to select useful variables for maximization of the pAUC.

The formulation of the pAUC is as follows. First, we fix the value of FPR in the range of $[\alpha_1, \alpha_2]$, where $\alpha_1 < \alpha_2$ and

$$\alpha_1 = \int \mathrm{H}(F(x_-) - c_1)g_-(x_-)dx_-, \quad \alpha_2 = \int \mathrm{H}(F(x_-) - c_2)g_-(x_-)dx_-.$$

The threshold values of c_1 and c_2 are determined so that the above equations hold. In practice, the pair ($\alpha_1 = 0, \alpha_2 = 0.1$) is often used. Then, the pAUC is given as

$$\mathrm{pAUC}(F, \alpha_1, \alpha_2) = \int_{c_1}^{c_2} \mathrm{TPR}(c)d\mathrm{FPR}(c)$$

$$= \int_{c_1}^{c_2} \left\{ \int_{c_2 \leq F(x_+) \leq c_1} \mathrm{H}(F(x_+) - c)g_+(x_+)dx_+ \right\} d\mathrm{FPR}(c) + \mathrm{TPR}(c_1)(\alpha_2 - \alpha_1).$$

The first term corresponds to the fan-shaped part of the pAUC; the other is the rectangular region below the fan-shaped part. Like the AUC, the pAUC has a probabilistic expression [25] as

$$\text{pAUC}(F, \alpha_1, \alpha_2) = P(F(X_+) \geq F(X_-), \ c_2 \leq F(X_-) \leq c_1).$$

Also, the surrogate pAUC is given as

$$\text{pAUC}_\sigma(F, \alpha_1, \alpha_2) = \int_{c_1}^{c_2} \left\{ \int_{c_2 \leq F(x_+) \leq c_1} \text{H}_\sigma(F(x_+) - c) g_+(x_+) dx_+ \right\} d\text{FPR}(c) + \text{TPR}(c_1)(\alpha_2 - \alpha_1)$$

satisfying

$$\sup_F \text{pAUC}_\sigma(F, \alpha_1, \alpha_2) = \text{pAUC}(\Lambda, \alpha_1, \alpha_2).$$

As learning machines, the authors of [22] consider the natural cubic splines for continuous variables and stumps for discrete variables, and demonstrate the utility of this approach based on gene expression data sets.

References

1. Bamber D (1975) The area above the ordinal dominance graph and the area below the receiver operating characteristic graph. J Math Psychol 12:387–415
2. Breiman L (2004) Population theory for boosting ensembles. Ann Stat 32:1–11
3. Chawla NV, Lazarevic A, Hall LO, Bowyer KW (2003) SMOTEBoost: improving prediction of the minority class in boosting. In: Lavrač N, Gamberger D, Todorovski L, Blockeel H (eds) Knowledge discovery in databases: PKDD 2003. Springer, Heidelberg, pp 107–119
4. Dettling M, Bühlmann P (2003) Boosting for tumor classification with gene expression data. Bioinformatics 19:1061–1069
5. Do JH, Choi D (2008) Clustering approaches to identifying gene expression patterns from DNA microarray data. Mol Cells 25:279–288
6. Dudoit S, Fridlyand J, Speed TP (2002) Comparison of discrimination methods for the classification of tumors using gene expression data. J Am Stat Assoc 97:77–87
7. Eguchi S, Copas J (2002) A class of logistic-type discriminant functions. Biometrika 89:1–22
8. Eisen MB, Spellman PT, Brown PO, Botstein D (1998) Cluster analysis and display of genome-wide expression patterns. Proc Natl Acad Sci U S A 95:14863–14868
9. Freund Y, Schapire RE (1997) A decision-theoretic generalization of on-line learning and an application to boosting. J Comput Syst Sci 55:119–139
10. Freund Y, Schapire RE (1999) A short introduction to boosting. J Jpn Soc Artif Intell 14:771–780
11. Friedman J (2002) Stochastic gradient boosting. Comput Stat Data Anal 38:367–378
12. Friedman J, Hastie T, Tibshirani R (2000) Additive logistic regression: a statistical view of boosting. Ann Stat 28:337–407
13. Fushiki T, Fujisawa H, Eguchi S (2006) Identification of biomarkers from mass spectrometry data using a "common" peak approach. BMC Bioinform 7:358
14. Galar M, Fernandez A, Barrenechea E, Bustince H, Herrera F (2012) A review on ensembles for the class imbalance problem: Bagging-, boosting-, and hybrid-based approaches. IEEE Trans Syst Man Cybern Part C (Applications and Reviews) 42:463–484

15. Golub TT, Slonim DK, Tamayo P, Huard C, Gaasenbeek M, Mesirov JP, Coller H, Loh ML, Downing JR, Caligiuri MA, Bloomfield CD, Lander ES (1999) Molecular classification of cancer: class discovery and class prediction by gene expression monitoring. Science 286:531–537

16. Hanley JA, McNeil BJ (1982) The meaning and use of the area under a receiver operating characteristic (ROC) curve. Radiology 143:29–36

17. Hastie T, Tibshirani R, Friedman J (2001) The elements of statistical learning: data mining, inference, and prediction. Springer, New York

18. Hastie T, Tibshirani R, Friedman J (2009) The elements of statistical learning: data mining, inference, and prediction, 2nd edn. Springer, New York

19. Joshi MV, Kumar V, Agarwal RC (2001) Evaluating boosting algorithms to classify rare classes: comparison and improvements. In: IBM research report, pp 1–20

20. Kawakita M, Minami M, Eguchi S, Lennert-Cody CE (2005) An introduction to the predictive technique AdaBoost with a comparison to generalized additive models. Fish Res 76:328–343

21. Komori O (2011) A boosting method for maximization of the area under the ROC curve. Ann Inst Stat Math 63:961–979

22. Komori O, Eguchi S (2010) A boosting method for maximizing the partial area under the ROC curve. BMC Bioinform 11:314

23. Lugosi BG, Vayatis N (2004) On the Bayes-risk consistency of regularized boosting methods. Ann Stat 32:30–55

24. Ma S, Huang J (2005) Regularized ROC method for disease classification and biomarker selection with microarray data. Bioinformatics 21:4356–4362

25. Pepe MS (2003) The statistical evaluation of medical tests for classification and prediction. Oxford University Press, New York

26. Pepe MS, Cai T, Longton G (2006) Combining predictors for classification using the area under the receiver operating characteristic curve. Biometrics 62:221–229

27. Pepe MS, Thompson ML (2000) Combining diagnostic test results to increase accuracy. Biostatistics 1:123–140

28. Schapire RE (1990) The strength of weak learnability. Mach Learn 5:197–227

29. Schapire RE, Freund Y, Bartlett P, Lee WS (1998) Boosting the margin: a new explanation for the effectiveness of voting methods. Ann Stat 26:1651–1686

30. Sørlie T, Perou CM, Tibshirani R, Aas T, Geisler S, Johnsen H, Hastie T, Eisen MB, van de Rijn M, Jeffrey SS, Thorsen T, Quist H, Matese JC, Brown PO, Botstein D, Lønning PE, Børresen-Dale A (2001) Gene expression patterns of breast carcinomas distinguish tumor subclasses with clinical implications. Proc Natl Acad Sci U S A 98:10869–10874

31. Takenouchi T, Ushijima M, Eguchi S (2007) GroupAdaBoost: accurate prediction and selection of important genes. IPSJ Digit Cour 3:145–152

32. van't Veer LJ, Dai H, van de Vijver MJ, He YD, Hart AAM, Mao M, Peterse HL, van der Kooy K, Marton MJ, Witteveen AT, Schreiber GJ, Kerkhoven RM, Roberts C, Linsley PS, Bernards R, Friend SH (2002) Gene expression profiling predicts clinical outcome of breast cancer. Nature 415:530–536

33. Wang Z, Chang YI, Ying Z, Zhu L, Yang Y (2007) A parsimonious threshold-independent protein feature selection method through the area under receiver operating characteristic curve. Bioinformatics 23:1794–2788

Appendix
Derivation of IC_β^b

For a dataset $D = \{x_1, \ldots, x_n\}$ and z, we define

$$L_D^b(\lambda) = -\sum_{i=1}^n \frac{\pi_\beta(x_i|\lambda)^b - 1}{b} + \frac{n}{1+b} \sum_{x \in \mathscr{X}} \pi_\beta(x|\lambda)^{1+b} \tag{A.1}$$

$$L_z^b(\lambda) = -\frac{\pi_\beta(z|\lambda)^b - 1}{b} + \frac{1}{1+b} \sum_{x \in \mathscr{X}} \pi_\beta(x|\lambda)^{1+b}, \tag{A.2}$$

where

$$\pi_\beta(x|\lambda) = \frac{\{1 + \beta\lambda^\top f(x)\}^{\frac{1}{\beta}}}{Z_\lambda} \tag{A.3}$$

and $Z_\lambda = \sum_{x \in \mathscr{X}} \{1 + \beta\lambda^\top f(x)\}^{1/\beta}$. Then, the estimator of λ is given as

$$\hat{\lambda}_\beta = \underset{\lambda}{\mathrm{argmin}} \, L_D^\beta(\lambda). \tag{A.4}$$

The bias term based on L_D^b is expressed as

$$\mathrm{bias}(G) = E_{G(D)}\Big[L_D^b(\hat{\lambda}_\beta) - n E_{G(z)}\{L_z^b(\hat{\lambda}_\beta)\}\Big], \tag{A.5}$$

where $G(D)$ and $G(z)$ are probability distribution of D and z, respectively. The term is divided into

$$\mathrm{bias}(G) = E_{G(D)}\Big[L_D^b(\hat{\lambda}_\beta) - L_D^b(\lambda_0)\Big] \tag{A.6}$$

$$+ E_{G(D)}\Big[L_D^b(\lambda_0) - n E_{G(z)}\{L_z^b(\lambda_0)\}\Big] \tag{A.7}$$

O. Komori and S. Eguchi, *Statistical Methods for Imbalanced Data in Ecological and Biological Studies*, JSS Research Series in Statistics,
https://doi.org/10.1007/978-4-431-55570-4

$$+ E_{G(D)} \left[n E_{G(z)} \{ L_D^b(\lambda_0) \} - n E_{G(z)} \{ L_z^b(\hat{\lambda}_\beta) \} \right] \quad \text{(A.8)}$$

$$\equiv D_1 + D_2 + D_3, \quad \text{(A.9)}$$

where $\lambda_0 = \text{argmin}_\lambda E_{G(z)}[L_z^\beta(\lambda)]$. Then we have

$$D_2 = E_{G(D)} \left[L_D^b(\lambda_0) - n E_{G(z)} \{ L_z^b(\lambda_0) \} \right] \quad \text{(A.10)}$$

$$= E_{G(D)} \{ L_D^b(\lambda_0) \} - n E_{G(z)} \{ L_z^b(\lambda_0) \} \quad \text{(A.11)}$$

$$= n E_{G(x_i)} \{ L_{x_i}^b(\lambda_0) \} - n E_{G(z)} \{ L_z^b(\lambda_0) \} \quad \text{(A.12)}$$

$$= 0 \quad \text{(A.13)}$$

because the observations $x_1, \ldots, x_n$ are independent. By Taylor expansion around λ_0, we have

$$E_{G(z)} \{ L_z^b(\hat{\lambda}_\beta) \} = E_{G(z)} \{ L_z^b(\lambda_0) \} + (\hat{\lambda}_\beta - \lambda_0)^\top E_{G(z)} \left[\left. \frac{\partial}{\partial \lambda} L_z^b(\lambda) \right|_{\lambda=\lambda_0} \right] \quad \text{(A.14)}$$

$$+ \frac{1}{2} (\hat{\lambda}_\beta - \lambda_0)^\top E_{G(z)} \left[\left. \frac{\partial^2}{\partial \lambda \partial \lambda^\top} L_z^b(\lambda) \right|_{\lambda=\lambda_0} \right] (\hat{\lambda}_\beta - \lambda_0) + o(n^{-1}). \quad \text{(A.15)}$$

Similarly, we have

$$L_D^b(\hat{\lambda}_\beta) = L_D^b(\lambda_0) + (\hat{\lambda}_\beta - \lambda_0)^\top \left. \frac{\partial}{\partial \lambda} L_D^b(\lambda) \right|_{\lambda=\lambda_0} \quad \text{(A.16)}$$

$$+ \frac{1}{2} (\hat{\lambda}_\beta - \lambda_0)^\top \left. \frac{\partial^2}{\partial \lambda \partial \lambda^\top} L_D^b(\lambda) \right|_{\lambda=\lambda_0} (\hat{\lambda}_\beta - \lambda_0) + o_p(1). \quad \text{(A.17)}$$

Note that

$$-\frac{1}{n} \left. \frac{\partial^2}{\partial \lambda \partial \lambda^\top} L_D^b(\lambda) \right|_{\lambda=\lambda_0} \xrightarrow{p} -E_{G(z)} \left[\left. \frac{\partial^2}{\partial \lambda \partial \lambda^\top} L_z^b(\lambda) \right|_{\lambda=\lambda_0} \right] \equiv J_b(\lambda_0). \quad \text{(A.18)}$$

Here we have

$$0 = \frac{1}{n} \left. \frac{\partial}{\partial \lambda} L_D^\beta(\lambda) \right|_{\lambda=\hat{\lambda}_\beta} \quad \text{(A.19)}$$

$$= \frac{1}{n} \left. \frac{\partial}{\partial \lambda} L_D^\beta(\lambda) \right|_{\lambda=\lambda_0} + (\hat{\lambda}_\beta - \lambda_0)^\top \frac{1}{n} \left. \frac{\partial^2}{\partial \lambda \partial \lambda^\top} L_D^\beta(\lambda) \right|_{\lambda=\lambda_0} + o_p(n^{-\frac{1}{2}}). \quad \text{(A.20)}$$

Hence we have

$$\hat{\lambda}_\beta - \lambda_0 = \left(-\frac{1}{n} \left. \frac{\partial^2}{\partial \lambda \partial \lambda^\top} L_D^\beta(\lambda) \right|_{\lambda=\lambda_0} \right)^{-1} \frac{1}{n} \left. \frac{\partial}{\partial \lambda} L_D^\beta(\lambda) \right|_{\lambda=\lambda_0} + o_p(n^{-\frac{1}{2}}). \text{ (A.21)}$$

Hence we have

$$D_1 + D_3 \tag{A.22}$$

$$= nE_{G(D)}\left[(\hat{\lambda}_\beta - \lambda_0)^\top\left\{\frac{1}{n}\frac{\partial}{\partial\lambda}L_D^b(\lambda)\bigg|_{\lambda=\lambda_0} - E_{G(z)}\left[\frac{\partial}{\partial\lambda}L_z^b(\lambda)\bigg|_{\lambda=\lambda_0}\right]\right\}\right] + o(1) \tag{A.23}$$

$$= nE_{G(D)}\left[-\frac{1}{n}\frac{\partial}{\partial\lambda}L_D^\beta(\lambda)\bigg|_{\lambda=\lambda_0}^\top J_\beta(\lambda_0)^{-1}\left\{\frac{1}{n}\frac{\partial}{\partial\lambda}L_D^b(\lambda)\bigg|_{\lambda=\lambda_0} - E_{G(z)}\left[\frac{\partial}{\partial\lambda}L_z^b(\lambda)\bigg|_{\lambda=\lambda_0}\right]\right\}\right] + o(1) \tag{A.24}$$

$$= n\text{tr}\left(J_\beta(\lambda_0)^{-1}E_{G(D)}\left[J_\beta(\lambda_0)^{-1}\left\{\frac{1}{n}\frac{\partial}{\partial\lambda}L_D^b(\lambda)\bigg|_{\lambda\lambda_0} - E_{G(z)}\left[\frac{\partial}{\partial\lambda}L_z^b(\lambda)\bigg|_{\lambda=\lambda_0}\right]\right\}\frac{1}{n}\frac{\partial}{\partial\lambda}L_D^\beta(\lambda)\bigg|_{\lambda=\lambda_0}^\top\right]\right) + o(1). \tag{A.25}$$

Here

$$E_{G(D)}\left[\frac{\partial}{\partial\lambda}L_D^b(\lambda)\bigg|_{\lambda=\lambda_0}\frac{\partial}{\partial\lambda}L_D^\beta(\lambda)\bigg|_{\lambda=\lambda_0}^\top\right] = nE_{G(z)}\left[\frac{\partial}{\partial\lambda}L_z^b(\lambda)\bigg|_{\lambda=\lambda_0}\frac{\partial}{\partial\lambda}L_z^\beta(\lambda)\bigg|_{\lambda=\lambda_0}^\top\right] \tag{A.26}$$

and

$$E_{G(D)}\left[\frac{\partial}{\partial\lambda}L_D^\beta(\lambda)\bigg|_{\lambda=\lambda_0}\right] = 0. \tag{A.27}$$

As a result, we have

$$\text{bias}(G) = D_1 + D_3 = \text{tr}\left(J_\beta(\lambda_0)^{-1}E_{G(z)}\left[\frac{\partial}{\partial\lambda}L_z^b(\lambda)\bigg|_{\lambda=\lambda_0}\frac{\partial}{\partial\lambda}L_z^\beta(\lambda)\bigg|_{\lambda=\lambda_0}^\top\right]\right) + o(1) \tag{A.28}$$

$$= \text{tr}\left(J_\beta(\lambda_0)^{-1}E_{G(z)}\left[\frac{\partial}{\partial\lambda}L_z^\beta(\lambda)\bigg|_{\lambda=\lambda_0}\frac{\partial}{\partial\lambda}L_z^b(\lambda)\bigg|_{\lambda=\lambda_0}^\top\right]\right) + o(1), \tag{A.29}$$

where $J_\beta(\lambda)$ is a symmetric matrix. Hence the corresponding estimator is

$$\text{bias}(\hat{G}) = \text{tr}\left(J_\beta(\hat{\lambda}_\beta)^{-1}\frac{1}{n}\sum_{i=1}^{n}\frac{\partial}{\partial\lambda}L_{x_i}^\beta(\lambda)\bigg|_{\lambda=\hat{\lambda}_\beta}\frac{\partial}{\partial\lambda}L_{x_i}^b(\lambda)\bigg|_{\lambda=\hat{\lambda}_\beta}^\top\right). \tag{A.30}$$

Hence the information criterion based on β-loss is given as

$$IC_\beta^b = 2\{L_D^b(\hat{\lambda}_\beta) - \text{bias}(\hat{G})\}, \tag{A.31}$$

which reduces to GIC when b goes to 0. The smaller value of IC_β^b means better estimation of λ_β.

Printed in the United States
By Bookmasters